CONTE

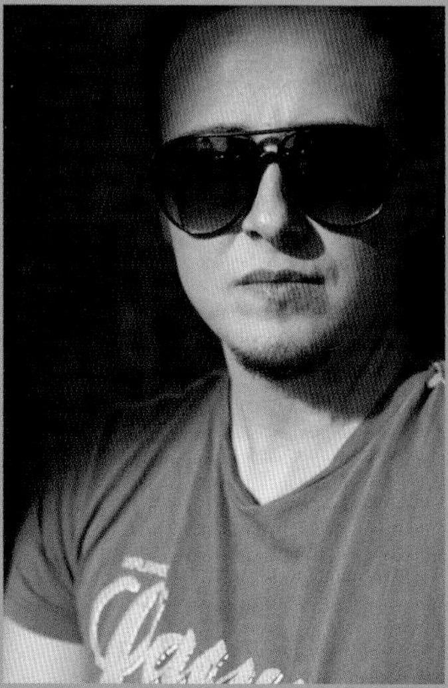

Written by Lee Gale & Dr Lewis Turner • Edited by Jim Pollard • Cartoons by Jason Barker • Photographs by Fox Fisher (plus Luke Stratta Photography and those pictured) • Advisory Board, chaired by Dr John Chisholm: Dr Richard Curtis, Alex Kaye, Jay McNeil, Bernard Reed, Terry Reed, Professor Stephen Whittle and Aeden Wolton • Thanks for the huge support from the community, to the many people who commented on drafts to ensure this publication is genuinely by us for us, and to all those who shared their photographs • Published: November 2015 • Revision date: November 2018

FOREWORD BY MARK REES

'Enjoy being a woman!' the lady psychiatrist purred as I was being discharged after several months as a mental patient. I wasn't 'mental', as we used to say then, just an undiagnosed transsexual. It was 1960 and life looked bleak but ten years later I was enabled to begin my transformation to Mark.

The medical world was waking up to the fact that we weren't psychotic. From then on, although treatment was patchy I was immensely relieved to be undergoing surgical and medical procedures that enabled me to live a happier life than ever envisaged. We owe much to the specialists who, in spite of the attitudes of some of their conservative colleagues and, of course, the press, continued with their efforts to ease the mental suffering of a misunderstood minority.

Now, many years later, the press plays little heed to us, even when we want it, and the public seems almost indifferent. Most of my journey, and I am sure contemporaries would agree, I 'played it by ear', which could be quite a lonely and confusing path. In all areas it seemed there were hurdles to surmount. It was a challenge but somehow we got there and perhaps consequently grew stronger.

Isolation and lack of information was then undoubtedly common to nearly everyone, both medics and folk in our situation. It is for that reason that I thoroughly applaud everyone who has been involved in the preparation of this excellent booklet. It will, I am sure, greatly ease and enhance the paths of those who are now setting out to what I hope will be a happy destination.

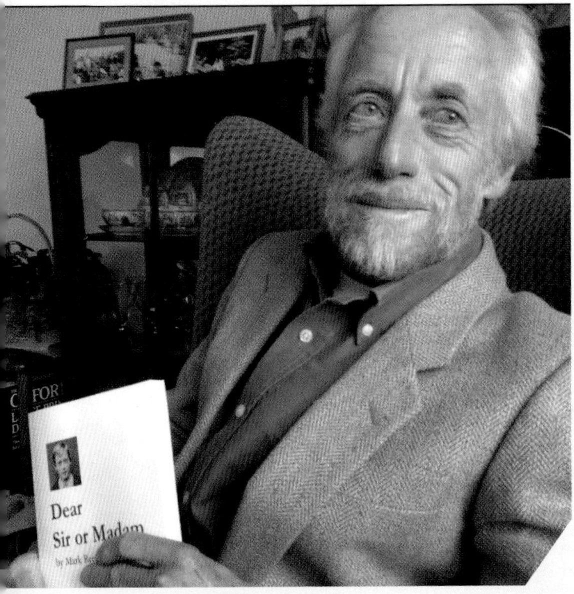

Mark Rees is a pioneer in gender transition who took the UK to the European Court of Human Rights in the 1980s because of its refusal to recognise his preferred gender in law. He tells his story in the acclaimed autobiography 'Dear Sir or Madam' (available in hardback from Mark at dsom@menshealthforum.org.uk or as ebook ISBN 978-0-9562734-1-3)

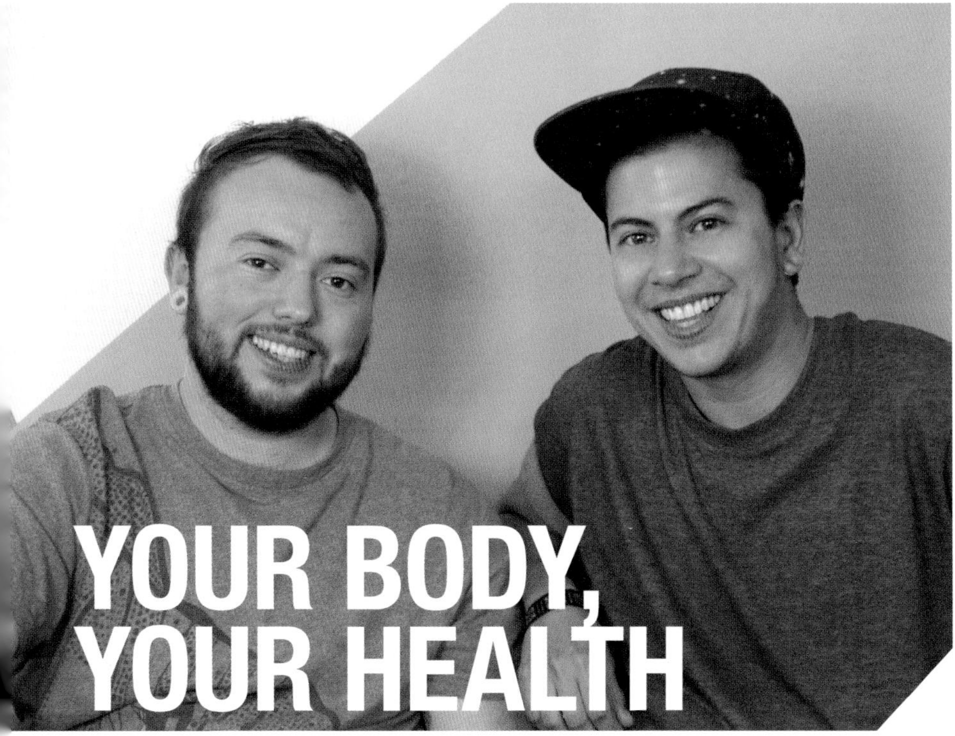

YOUR BODY, YOUR HEALTH

WHO IS THIS GUIDE FOR?

It's for anyone who thinks they might find it useful.

Specifically, it is aimed at people who were registered as (assigned) female at birth (AFAB), and who are moving (transitioning) or are interested in moving towards a male or more masculine identity or presentation. This includes, but is not limited to, man, trans man, trans* man, trans masculine, non-binary, masculine of centre, androgynous, boi, gender fluid and genderqueer identities.

We have thought long and hard about how we can be inclusive in this guide and make it easier to read and have decided to use the term 'trans man' as a shorthand to include all of these identities. Even though it may not explicitly describe your identity, you are still included.

The guide will be useful to people of all ages. There are many more young people questioning their gender identity at a much earlier age, some as young as three or four years old and parents of these children may also find it useful to know what services and support are available.

Above all, the guide is written for trans men by trans men. It explains the various aspects of transition healthcare and provides the information you need to help you make decisions about your own wellbeing and deal with the challenges you might encounter when dealing with a health care system (and wider society) which can still tend to think in terms of two fixed genders.

THE WORDS WE USE

Language is both very important and very individual. We each have words that we like to use and words we don't feel comfortable with or even hate.

Language within trans communities is developing and the same word can mean different things to different people.

When writing this guide, we have tried to use words sensitively and be aware of how the language may make people feel. We have tried to be as inclusive and as clear as possible and to use medical terminology where needed (and to avoid placing gender on these words) so that we're clear about what is being discussed.

You may not identify with all of the language used here, but we hope that it is still accessible to you and you feel able to take the information you need from it.

The NHS uses the term gender dysphoria, 'which is a condition where a person experiences discomfort or distress because there is a mismatch between their biological sex and gender identity'.

YOUR BODY, YOUR CHOICE

Please take from this guide whatever you want. There are lots of links to further information and support.

But remember this isn't a checklist for how to transition. That doesn't exist. It's entirely up to you to decide what is important for you.

This guide aims to give you information on the possibilities but this doesn't mean that you have to go through all these steps or procedures or that you have to do them in a certain order or even that you have to do any of them at all. The information is here if you need it.

Try not to rush into decisions now, especially if you're unsure, as it's much harder to reverse the process if it turns out not to be right for you. You can always change your mind in the future and go ahead with something later if it becomes important to you.

Take responsibility for your life and your needs. It's up to you to tell people what you need and what's important to you, so be honest with yourself and with medical professionals.

LOOK AFTER YOUR BODY

This guide doesn't just give information on options for transition, but also on general wellbeing and lifestyle. For some of us it can be hard to acknowledge our bodies or to look after them. Some of us can feel angry and may try to punish ourselves and our bodies. However, looking after your health and body as best you can will have many benefits. You will have more energy, your mental health will improve and you'll find the stresses you may face easier to deal with.

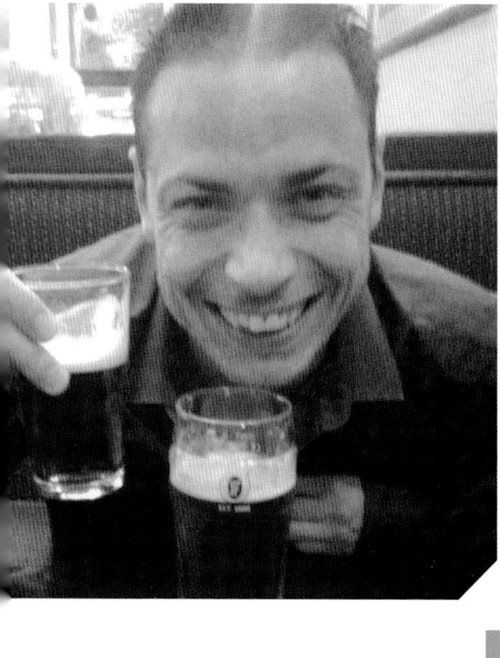

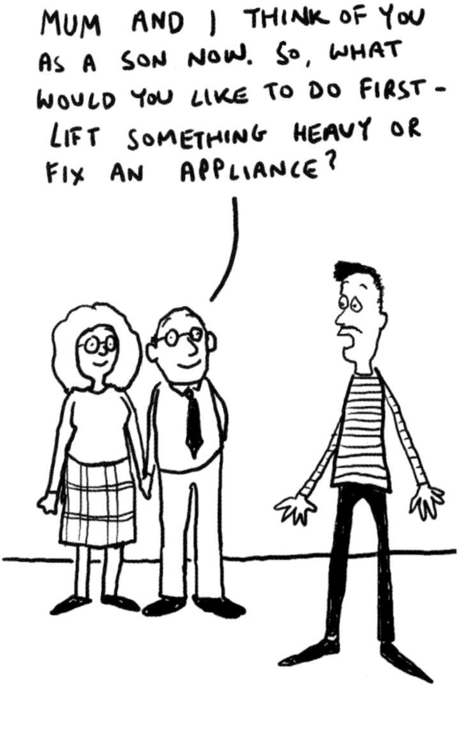

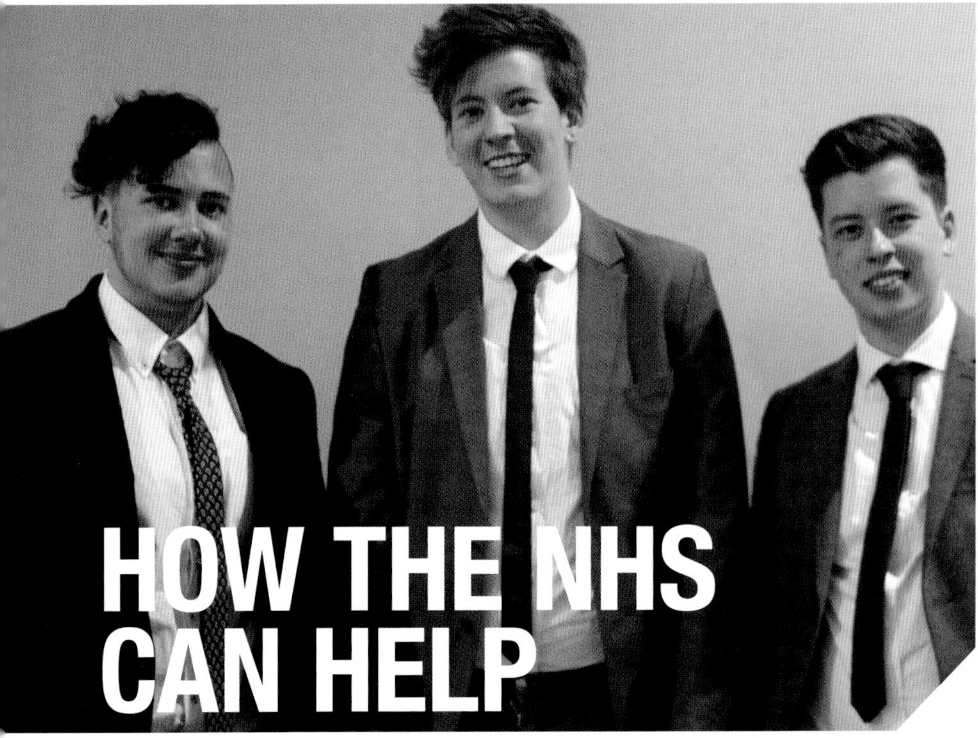

HOW THE NHS CAN HELP

If you want to change your body, there are a number of options – some big, some small. The NHS can help with many of them with different support at different ages. Some services will be limited until you're older, but you can still access lots of information and support.

The NHS is available to all people in the UK who are 'ordinarily resident' which means that you are living in the UK legally and on a 'properly settled basis' for the time being. Details of what this means and what you can access if you're not resident can be found on the NHS website. Follow the Men's Health Forum website link in the Further Information section on page 65.

CAN I GET MEDICAL HELP?

Yes. To help us feel more comfortable in our bodies and to help others see us for who we are, it is possible for trans people to medically transition (get medical treatment) on the NHS or through a private route. This guide concentrates on the NHS options.

People make decisions based on many things including what they feel they need, their relationship with their body, cultural or religious influences and what they can physically or financially cope with. Take your time to make these decisions and find out as much as you can before you go ahead. Some people like to read about the options and/or to speak to people who have already gone through a medical transition.

HOW DO I ACCESS SERVICES?

For everyone who wants or needs to get help from the NHS and is aged 18 or over, the first place to go is to your local doctor (the general practitioner or GP). Tell them about how you feel and that you'd like a referral to one of the specialist gender services or Gender Identity Clinics (GIC).

In England you are able to choose which one you'd prefer to go to. Some clinics have longer waiting times than others and you may have to wait up to a year or even longer before you get your first appointment.

Information for under 18s is on page 12.

WHAT IF MY GP ISN'T FAMILIAR WITH TRANS ISSUES?

Few GPs know a lot about trans issues unless they already have patients who are trans, but that doesn't mean they won't be supportive or willing to educate themselves. Many GPs are very supportive but on occasion you might find that your GP doesn't know how to refer you or may even refuse to help you.

It is important to find a GP who is supportive, as they will help you through the process and will have a role in your care. If you want to medically transition, you may need your GP to write referral letters for surgery, prescribe you hormones and do regular blood tests.

If your GP seems supportive and willing to learn, point them in the right direction. There are lots of resources and information they can access to inform themselves. The charity GIRES, in conjunction with the Royal College of GPs, have developed an e-learning resource for GPs – details in the Further Information section on page 65.

If you find that your GP isn't willing to help you or you feel uncomfortable with them, then find a new one (see page 58). This could be another doctor in the same practice or a doctor in a different practice if you have another surgery nearby.

WHERE ARE THE UK'S GENDER IDENTITY CLINICS?

There are seven Gender Identity Clinics (GICs) across England. You'll need a referral from a GP to these clinics and can choose which one you'd like to attend:

> London
> Sheffield
> Leeds
> Northumberland
> Northampton
> Nottingham
> Exeter.

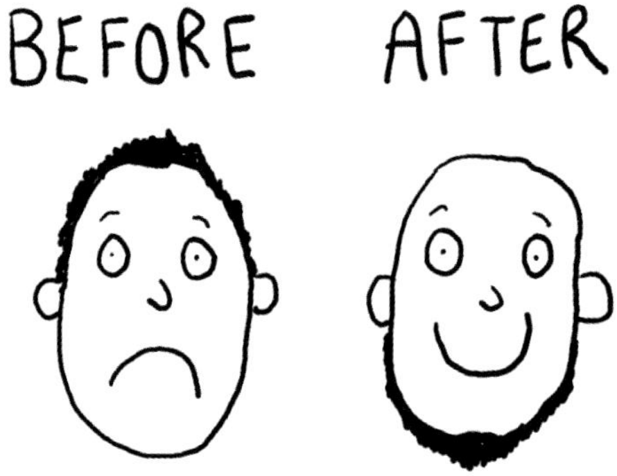

There are four in Scotland. You can self-refer to some of these:

> Glasgow
> Edinburgh (only accept in area referrals)
> Inverness (only accept in area referrals)
> Aberdeen (only accept in area referrals).

There is one GIC in Northern Ireland based in Belfast while those seeking referral from Wales are currently sent to London.

Check page 66 for the full addresses of each clinic.

WHAT SERVICES ARE AVAILABLE FROM THE NHS?

There are many options for treatment and support available from the NHS and it's up to you which ones you decide to have and which ones you decide aren't necessary for you. It's also OK to change your mind if you decide you do want some form of treatment a few months or even a few years later. You can access hormone treatment, affirmation (reassignment) surgery and in some clinics psychological support (talking to people about how you feel).

There are sections in this guide which go into these in more detail. The section on hormones is on page 13; the section on chest surgery options is on page 22 and the section on options down below on page 27.

YOUR FIRST GENDER IDENTITY CLINIC APPOINTMENT

Make sure you're comfortable. There's no need to dress in a certain way or style, wear whatever makes you feel confident and able to speak about yourself.

You may want to take some supporting information along with you, such as:

> a name change document (if you have one, but don't worry if you don't),

> a list of medication or other health products that you're on

> any letters or documents relating to previous treatment (if you have any)

> any information that supports your intention to transition, such as letters of support

It might also be useful to take:

> a written history in case you forget to make a point that you feel is important

> a list of any questions you have or points that you want to talk about, again so you don't forget, and

> any other gender-related documentation you have changed such as deed poll/statutory declaration for name change, driving licence or passport.

Most services allow you to take someone with you to support you. It also helps to have another pair of ears there to remember things that have been discussed. Feel free to take notes too, if that helps.

WHAT TO EXPECT AT YOUR FIRST APPOINTMENT

Different clinics across the UK work in slightly different ways, but at all of them you'll have to go through an initial assessment. This could involve two to six appointments (depending on the clinic) as in most places they like you to see a couple of different clinicians.

The specialist will probably want to ask questions about your history. These can include questions around how you felt as a child, your relationships with your family, how you feel about your body and about other relationships you may have had. They're not trying to trip you up or make you feel uncomfortable, they're just trying to get to know you a bit better. It might seem quite personal and some of the questions might feel uncomfortable for you. If it does, then let them know, but be honest with them about how you feel.

WHAT IS MEANT BY REAL LIFE EXPERIENCE (RLE)?

You might have come across people talking about having to do an RLE before you can access certain treatments. This is a period of time in which, in the words of the NHS, someone is expected to be 'living in the gender role that is congruent with an individual's gender identity'. This means that you are expected to live according to the gender role and expression (how you dress, for instance) that feels right for you. It includes things like changing your name and documents and coming out to friends, family, colleagues or classmates.

In the NHS guidelines, it states that before you can access genital surgery you must have been living 'in role' for 12-24 months. Before accessing chest surgery, you must have started this process, but you don't need to have completed it. How all this is interpreted can vary in different gender clinics.

I'M 17 OR UNDER, CAN I STILL ACCESS SERVICES FROM THE NHS?

Yes, people of all ages are able to access gender services on the NHS. Some of the adult clinics listed above will see people from 17 – see the list of clinics on page 66.

If you are under 18, you can be referred to a specialist service called Gender Identity Development Services (GIDS) at the Tavistock and Portman Clinic. Their main clinic is in London, but they also have a small clinic based in Leeds and another in Exeter. There is also a service in Scotland called the Sandyford Clinic in Glasgow and one in Northern Ireland called Knowing Our Identity based in Belfast. These services will help you to explore your gender identity and expression and can also work with your family and help them understand what you're experiencing.

You can be referred to the service through your GP, social services, education departments, your school nurse or your local Child and Adolescent Mental Health Service (CAMHS), which you can access by going to your GP. Although you or your family can't make a direct referral, you can contact the clinic for information on referrals.

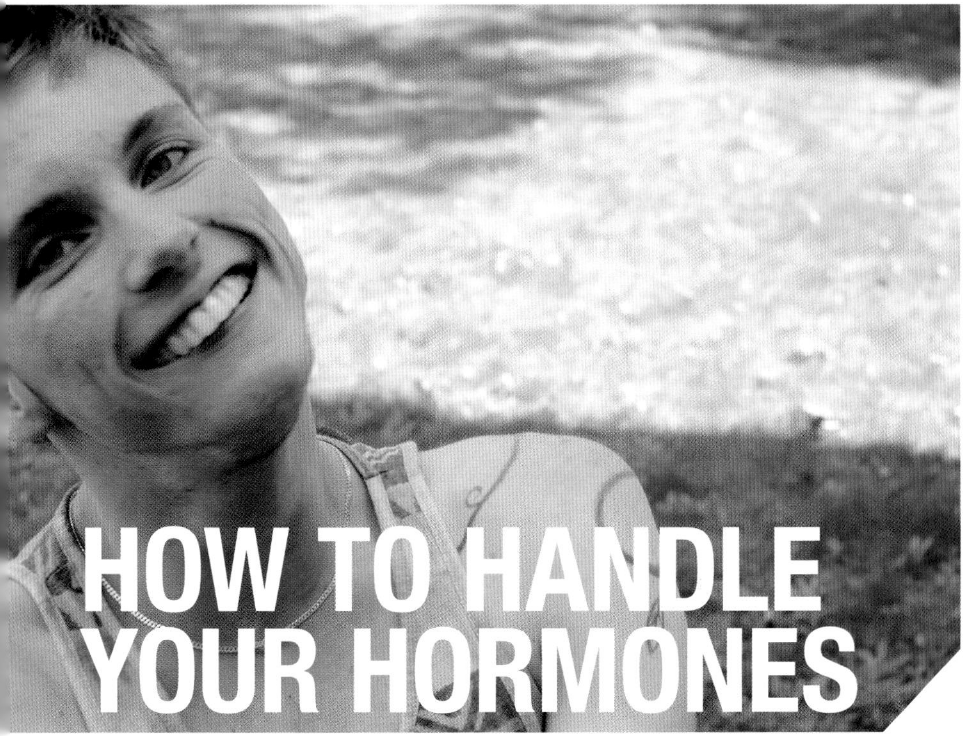

HOW TO HANDLE YOUR HORMONES

Hormones are the body's chemical messengers. They are key to how you look and feel. This sections tells you all you need to know about hormones.

WHAT IS TESTOSTERONE?

Testosterone is the most important masculinising hormone (although people assigned female at birth also produce it at a lower level)

If you start testosterone hormone replacement therapy (HRT) you will go through the sort of puberty that those assigned male at birth experience, which will bring about physical changes.

You will need to be on testosterone throughout your life. You need some form of hormone therapy particularly if you are to have your ovaries removed as it may help prevent brittle bones (osteoporosis).

HOW DO I TAKE TESTOSTERONE?

There are different ways to take testosterone and after a few years, people usually find a way which suits them.

Sustanon 250mg, which is the testosterone hormone-replacement therapy specifically licensed for trans men, is given as an injection every 2-3 weeks. Sustanon is suspended in peanut oil.

Other injectable forms of HRT include Testosterone Enanthate 250mg (which is suspended in castor oil if you are allergic to peanuts and also given every 2-3 weeks) or Nebido 1g (injected every 10-14 weeks.)

These are intramuscular injections – usually in your bottom or thigh. Some trans men get a nurse at their GP surgery to do this; some do it themselves.

I DON'T LIKE THE IDEA OF INJECTIONS

Injections can be stressful. If the injection is in the right place (always ask a nurse to show you where), you may well feel some minor pain for a short period of time. In the long-term, injections may wear you down a bit. It can help with injecting Nebido if you warm up the ampoule in some hot water.

WHAT ARE THE ALTERNATIVES?

There is gel with brand names like Testim (in tubes), Tostran (in a pump container) and Testogel (in sachets). Gel is applied to the skin daily. But cover up if cuddling other people just after applying the gel as it can be transferred!

Many people are quite happy with gel but we're all different and some have found that gel may not be enough to 'kickstart' puberty. If you're not sure the method you're using is right for you, discuss it with your specialist but try not to be too impatient and give it a few months.

I AM 10 YEARS OLD – CAN I STOP MY BODY GOING THROUGH A FEMALE PUBERTY?

If you are under the care of the Sandyford Clinic, Tavistock and Portman GIDS or Knowing Our Identity (see page 66), they may wait until the first signs of puberty (this depends not on age but stage of development) and prescribe you with Goserelin or Leuprorelin which are 'blockers'. This is a subcutaneous (under the skin) injection which suspends puberty. This puberty can be resumed if you change your mind but if your gender identity remains the same by the age of 16 you can then be prescribed testosterone.

CAN YOU BUY HORMONES ON THE INTERNET?

Yes – if you have a prescription. To sell drugs online legally in the UK, a company must be registered with the Medicines and Healthcare products Regulatory Agency (MHRA). No MHRA-registered company will sell you drugs without a prescription. So if you don't have a prescription, get one.

Do not buy from sites that will sell you hormones without a prescription. They are unregulated and illegal and you really don't know what you are going to be sold. If you cannot wait until you get hormones on the NHS consider going private as this will be safer.

WHAT WILL HAPPEN WHEN I START HORMONES?

You will begin to experience symptoms of the menopause (if you have ovaries) as well as puberty at the same time, which can have many effects on your body and how you feel.

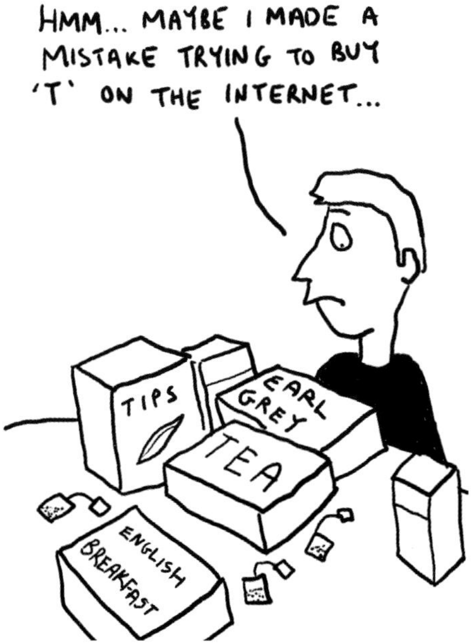

Your periods usually stop after around five months but it can take longer – don't worry. If they have not stopped after six months your levels may need adjusting. You may notice changes in your voice – usually beginning with a sore throat, which is the first sign of your voice breaking. You might develop acne on your back, neck and your face – if so, talk to your pharmacist or GP about ways to control this.

Remember, this is a second puberty so you may feel more inclined to do more risky things and might overestimate what you can handle.

Don't forget your age – you may be mistaken for a teenage boy, but if you are 35 you should have the wisdom of your age!

For your first 18 months on testosterone you may find that you sweat a lot more than usual – especially the first summer. This usually passes.

IF MY PERIODS STOP, I DON'T NEED TO HAVE SMEAR TESTS, RIGHT?

Wrong. You still need to have smear tests if you are over 25 years old as long as you have a cervix.

If or when you change your gender marker on your medical records, you will no longer be automatically notified of when to have a smear test. It is then your responsibility to schedule them.

WHAT HAPPENS IF I TAKE MORE TESTOSTERONE THAN PRESCRIBED?

This is not a good idea because any excess testosterone will be converted by your body to oestrogen (feminising hormones) which you don't want. It will also make your blood thicker, cause you to put on more subcutaneous fat and raise your risk of pulmonary embolism (blocked artery), a deep vein thrombosis or a stroke. Also see long term effects on page 20.

WHAT IF I WANT OR NEED A LOWER DOSE OF TESTOSTERONE?

The changes that occur are mostly to do with your genetics and not to do with the dosage you take. But some people may want a lower dose of testosterone because of their health or because of the way they identify.

It is impossible to tightly control the type or amount of changes that you get. Some people who have experimented with lower dosages have found that they experience slower changes, but this won't be the case for everyone.

Hormones are really important and play a part in maintaining many different functions of the body. Having lower doses of testosterone may risk impairing some of these functions. Always make sure that your treatment is overseen by your GP and, if necessary, an endocrinologist. Work with your doctor(s) to ensure you're as safe as possible.

WHAT ABOUT SEX DRIVE?

You may notice you are regularly thinking about sex – sometimes for no reason at all. It can be distracting but usually calms down after around 18-24 months.

WILL TESTOSTERONE MAKE ME MORE AGGRESSIVE?

Not necessarily. Many people report being less aggressive than they were before – possibly because they feel happier in themselves – although some report that they feel less able to cry.

IS IT TRUE THAT YOU GROW A SMALL PENIS?

Not really. Your clitoris will begin to grow – it will develop a 'helmet' like a penis has and will become very sensitive for a while. You might have to buy some looser fitting underwear to make yourself more comfortable.

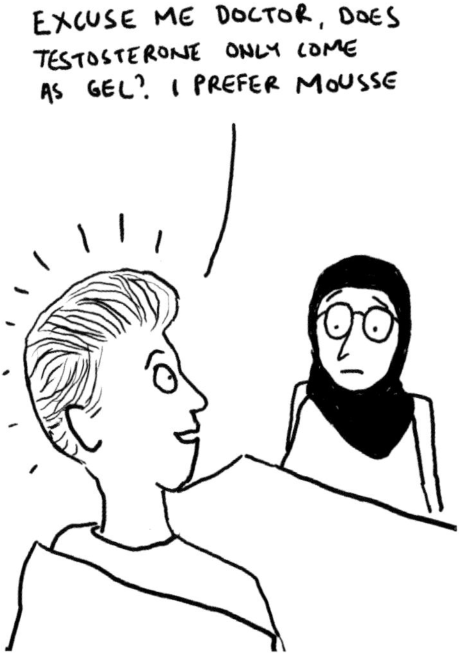

How big it grows depends on these things called 'androgen receptors' we have in the tissues in our bodies.

Some of us have more androgen receptors in the tissue of our clitoris than others. It is just down to genetics. Maximum growth is usually reached after around two years.

WILL I GROW BIG MUSCLES?

This is down to genetics. Everyone is different. If you have a body type that puts on muscle easily at the moment then, if you work out regularly over a long period of time, you will. But some people don't have that kind of build at all.

WILL I LOSE FAT FROM MY HIPS?

Testosterone changes the fat distribution around your body. The fat usually moves from the hips to the stomach (where it can be more dangerous). Some people don't get rid of all the fat from their hips – again this is down to genetics and 'androgen receptors'. It is important to remember that many people assigned male at birth have fat on their hips as well.

WILL MY BODY GET BIGGER ANYWAY?

You will notice an increase in your appetite. Some notice that they have put on weight and it can make them depressed as well as cause problems when they want surgery. Don't stop eating to try and lose fat as your body will immediately start to retain calories. It is better to eat healthily and take regular exercise. (See the section on page 48 for tips on healthy eating and exercise.)

Don't rush to buy loads of new clothes when you start testosterone. You will find that your body changes don't settle down for around two years and it will be expensive to change your whole wardrobe several times.

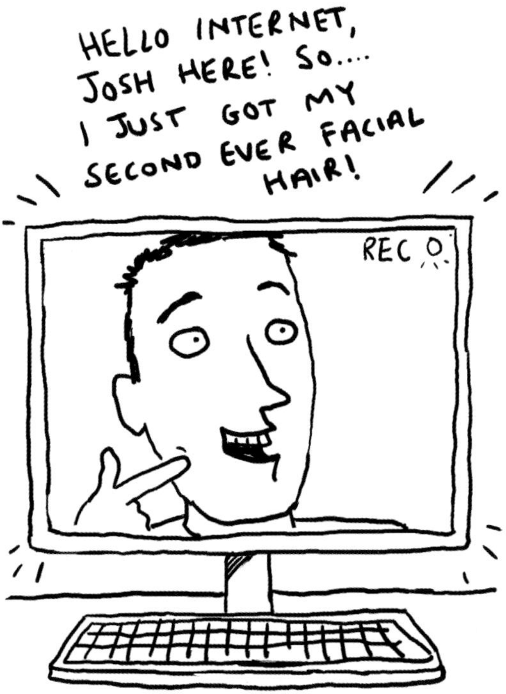

CAN I GET PREGNANT IF TAKING TESTOSTERONE?

Yes, possibly even in the absence of periods.

WILL I GROW A BEARD?

It all depends on genetics, ethnicity and 'androgen receptors'. Some people have thicker beard growth than others – and some have very little facial hair. You will just have to wait and see as it can take up to ten years for facial hair to thicken. You may also see an increase in body hair.

WILL I GO BALD?

Again, it is all down to the genes in your family and those 'androgen receptors'. If you do start to go bald, there is nothing you can do to stop it.

WHAT ELSE SHOULD I WATCH OUT FOR PHYSICALLY?

Some experience strange cramps – very similar to period pain – which can continue for a few years on and off. Don't worry, this is simply the testosterone's effects on your ovaries and womb and usually disappears once everything has settled down. If it doesn't, you should consider having a hysterectomy.

You may also experience hot flushes for the first year on testosterone. Physical exercise can help with reducing pain and hot flushes. Some people report that drinking nettle tea can reduce hot flushes.

There is a possibility, with testosterone therapy, of changes to the number of red blood cells in the blood (polycythaemia), the thyroid gland, the liver or the pituitary gland. All of these can cause itching. This usually settles down but if it continues for more than six months, ask for a referral to an endocrinologist to discuss it.

WHAT ABOUT NEGATIVE EFFECTS ON MOOD?

You may find you have mood swings as well. You might feel on top of the world about the changes one minute and then a bit overwhelmed about everything the next. Some trans men who take hormones via an injection say that they feel more moody for 3-4 days afterwards. Check out the section on page 43 for some tips on looking after yourself.

Communication is key to making sure that everybody understands what is happening, and you need to find yourself a personal space to go to when you feel low. Some go to the gym or go running at this point as they find the natural endorphins of exercise help them.

WHAT'S THE EFFECT ON OTHER HEALTH CONDITIONS?

Many trans men have experienced mental health challenges before hormones and some will continue to be treated once they have started them. For some, gender dysphoria and depression are two separate issues.

Some people who are already on the autistic spectrum may find that their autistic tendencies can be enhanced by testosterone. Others have found that testosterone can worsen symptoms of Obsessive Compulsive Disorder.

Like any changes in hormones, taking testosterone can also trigger epilepsy for a very small minority.

ANY LONG TERM EFFECTS OF TESTOSTERONE?

There has not been much research in this area, but evidence suggests that the life expectancy of a trans man on testosterone is the same as anyone assigned male at birth. True, life expectancy of those assigned male at birth is shorter than those assigned female, but lifestyle factors like smoking play a bigger role in life expectancy than gender.

However, testosterone causes changes inside your body as well as the outside. It will increase cholesterol giving you a higher risk of heart disease as cholesterol can clog your arteries. There are often no symptoms for high cholesterol which is why it's a good idea to keep an eye on your weight and not smoke.

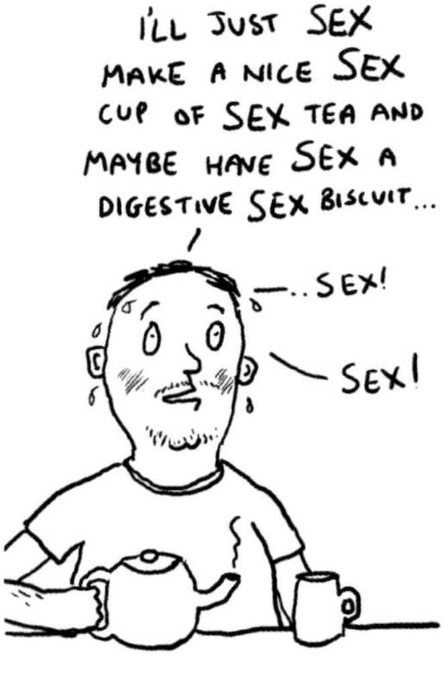

Testosterone also increases the number of red blood cells – making your blood 'thicker' meaning that you can get blood clots a lot easier which can cause a stroke. This is why you need regular blood checks from your doctor.

WHAT BLOOD TESTS DO I NEED FROM MY GP?

Your GP should test these every six months for the first two years, then yearly: blood pressure, full blood count, thyroid, urea and electrolytes, liver function tests, fasting glucose, lipid profile, testosterone and oestrogen.

WHAT IS THE IDEAL TESTOSTERONE LEVEL?

There isn't one. The ideal level will be different for one person compared to another. Ultimately, the best level is the lowest dose that you feel comfortable with. (Remember that so-called normal levels in the UK are based on white British men.)

WHICH RED BLOOD CELL LEVEL APPLIES TO ME?

If you're taking testosterone, you may wonder which red blood cell count level is right for you – male or female. The experts don't know the answer to this as not enough research has been done. If your red blood cell count is very high, it is called polycythemia. If you smoke, stop because smoking raises your red blood cell count anyway

If you have polycythemia, you should see a specialist endocrinologist. It may be improved by switching from testosterone injections to gel. If this still does not resolve your blood cell count you may need to have some blood taken from your body (venesection).

WHAT ELSE SHOULD I WATCH OUT FOR?

You should consider having occasional ankle bone scans to check for osteoporosis – brittle bone disease.

Regularly check your chest – even after surgery. A small amount of breast tissue remains after chest reconstruction surgery and therefore breast cancer is still a possibility in the same way that all men have a risk of breast cancer, so checking for lumps is important.

You should also have your blood pressure checked regularly.

WHAT WOULD HAPPEN IF I CAME OFF TESTOSTERONE AFTER A FEW YEARS?

The consequences of stopping testosterone depend on several factors such as the length of time on treatment, the extent of masculinisation and whether or not you've had a hysterectomy.

Some people who have not had a hysterectomy have found that their periods started again. But others have found that they are now infertile. Most of the effects of testosterone are reversible but the body hair and the voice will not revert to how they were before.

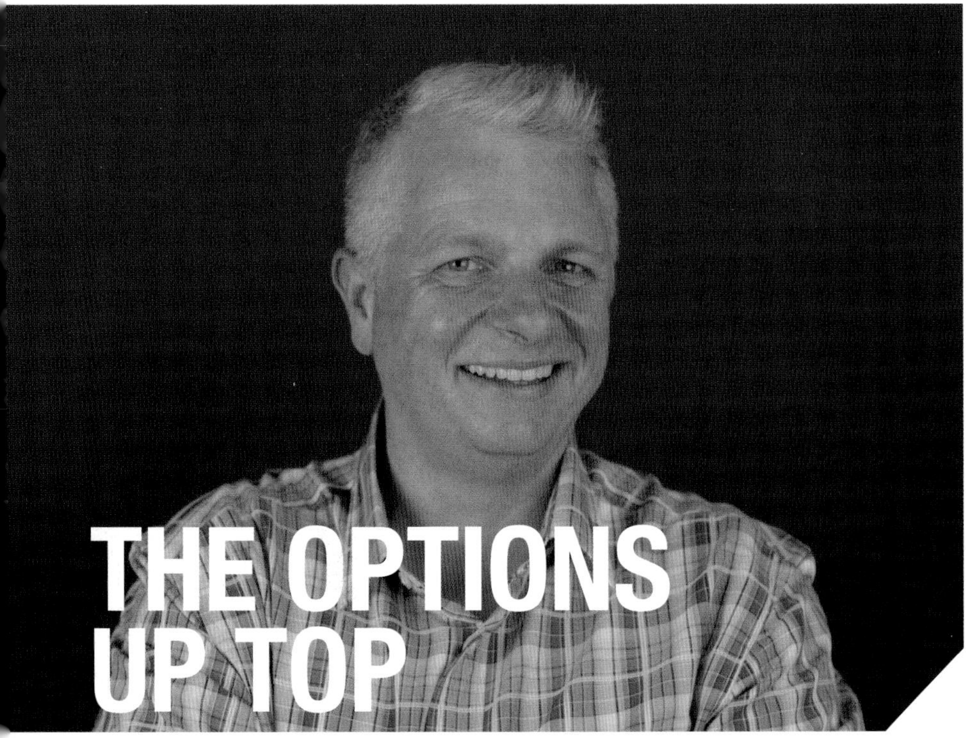

THE OPTIONS UP TOP

There are a number of things you can do to change how your chest looks and feels. This section covers the surgical and non-surgical options.

WHAT DOES CHEST BINDING DO?

It compresses the chest and makes it appear flatter. You can get binders online (look up 'compression shirts'). Many trans men use companies such as Underworks, Gc2b and Peecock.

The best one depends on your size and what works for you. People who don't have a lot up top sometimes use sports bras. Shop around and see what is being said on online forums. There are also binder exchange schemes within some trans men's groups like MORF.

ARE BINDERS SAFE TO WEAR?

It is not good if your binder is so tight that it affects your breathing. There are also risks to wearing a tight binder for too long: bruised or fractured ribs, back and other muscular-skeletal problems, damage to tissue and blood vessels round the chest, blood clots and loss of sensation around the chest area. It is better if you only wear it for a few hours in the day and not over many years. You should never sleep in your binder.

ACE/Crepe bandages are not safe as they constrict over time and can cause long term health problems as well as affect surgery results.

WHAT ARE MY OPTIONS FOR TOP SURGERY?

There are three main options in the UK for top surgery and depend on the surgeon's technique and/or what is most appropriate for your chest size.

SURGERY FOR SMALLER CHESTS

Option 1: Liposuction

This is for those who have not really developed as much. The fat around the chest is sucked out. There will usually only be small scars under the armpits and the tips of the nipples may need to be 'shaved'.

Option 2: Keyhole/Peri areolar incision

An incision is made all the way around the areola (the darker skin around the nipple), removing a doughnut of skin and the breast tissue is removed, usually leaving the areola attached to maintain blood and nerve supply. The remaining skin is then pulled in and stitched to the areola leaving a scar only around the areola, which is usually well hidden.

For smaller chests, an incision can be made only part way round the areola, breast tissue removed, and the skin left to retract afterwards. For larger chests, a modified peri-areolar technique can sometimes be used that produces scars that extend out from the areolae.

What's good?

The advantage for both of these methods is that there is minimal scarring and more chance of maintaining nipple sensation.

What's not so good?

It can be more difficult to produce a smooth looking chest by peri-areolar techniques, so there is a risk of a lumpy or dented appearance.Some trans men have experienced nipple loss and others experience swelling which can take several months to go down.

SURGERY FOR LARGER CHESTS

Double incision

In this method, two long horizontal cuts are made across the chest. The breast tissue is then removed along with any excess skin and the nipples may be repositioned if necessary.

What's good?

It is the best result for people who are bigger. The scars usually follow the contours of the chest muscle and in time may not be prominent (although some individuals retain thick red scars). This method gives a more immediate cosmetic result as less time is needed for skin retraction which occurs after the peri-arelor technique.

What's not so good?

The disadvantage is that there is more scarring and there may be excess skin around the scar – 'dog ears'. However, these can be worked on at a later date – called a 'revision'. There may be loss of sensation in the nipples and some trans men lose their nipples (but you can achieve very realistic nipples through tattoos). If you have darker skin you are more likely to get keloid scars – talk with the surgeon about the risks.

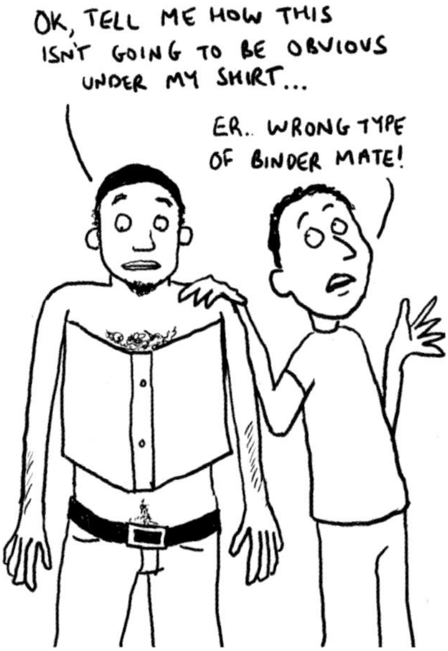

WHAT ABOUT POST-OP CARE?

You may have drains (very thin tubes) in your chest for excess blood and fluid. You will have to return to the surgeon after a couple of days to have these removed and perhaps stitches too. A binder may be needed for four weeks after to compress the chest. The surgeon will give you instructions on how long until you can exercise again and how long you need to take off work.

Some people recommend using the fluid in vitamin E capsules or Bio Oil to help the scars heal.

You may experience keloid scarring, which are large lumpy scars. They can be helped by compression to flatten the scar in conjunction with a silicone-based scar treatment such as Kelo Kote gel and Mepiform sheets.

If it is severe, you can ask your GP for a referral to a dermatologist for steroid injections into the scar.

WHAT SHOULD I TAKE TO HOSPITAL FOR TOP SURGERY?

> pyjama tops – ensure that they have buttons going down the front as you will probably be unable to raise your arms.

> loose fitting shirts with buttons down the front

> a wash bag containing toiletries, including your toothbrush and toothpaste

> tracksuit bottoms or shorts/trousers with elasticated waist

> pillow for protecting chest from seat belt if you are returning home by car after surgery

> post-op binder

> phone charger and mobile phone.

> books, magazines etc.

WHEN CAN I TAKE MY TOP OFF IN THE SUN?

Usually you'll be advised to keep scars protected from the sun for a year to allow the scars to heal – so cover up or use high factor (50+) sun block to protect scars when you do take your top off.

I'VE HAD TOP SURGERY AND I DON'T THINK THEY TOOK ENOUGH AWAY

This is quite a common reaction after liposuction or keyhole/peri-areola techniques as it may not give you a completely flat chest. Look around at other guys who are not trans – very few have completely flat chests unless they are very skinny. You can return to your surgeon within a year of the surgery to discuss the possibility of a revision if you are not happy.

You might want to build up your upper chest muscles (pectorals) a bit, around six months after surgery, by doing press-ups at home or bench press exercises in the gym. This will help get a bit more shape.

WHICH SURGEON SHOULD I CHOOSE?

Surgeons can only work with the body tissue that each individual has so you cannot expect a surgeon to give the same results for everyone. Do your research – there are some online groups who do a 'show and tell' for different surgeons and there may be some they recommend. It is important that you feel comfortable with the surgeon as well as confident in their ability.

IS IT A GOOD IDEA TO LOSE WEIGHT BEFORE SURGERY?

Yes it is because you are likely to get a better result as there will be less for the surgeon to remove. If you are very overweight, a surgeon may ask you to lose weight before they operate.

WHAT ARE THE RISKS?

Any surgery has its risks and your surgeon will discuss these with you. Some trans men have found that after top surgery, they have numbness or shooting pain in their chest for years to come or tingling in the arms or round the scar.

CAN TRANS MEN GET BREAST CANCER AFTER TOP SURGERY?

The risk of breast cancer is not reduced from having top surgery, as not all breast tissue is removed so you should still check your chest for lumps.

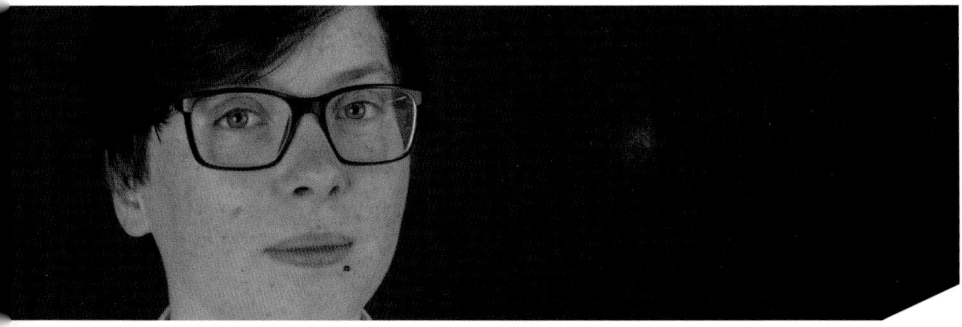

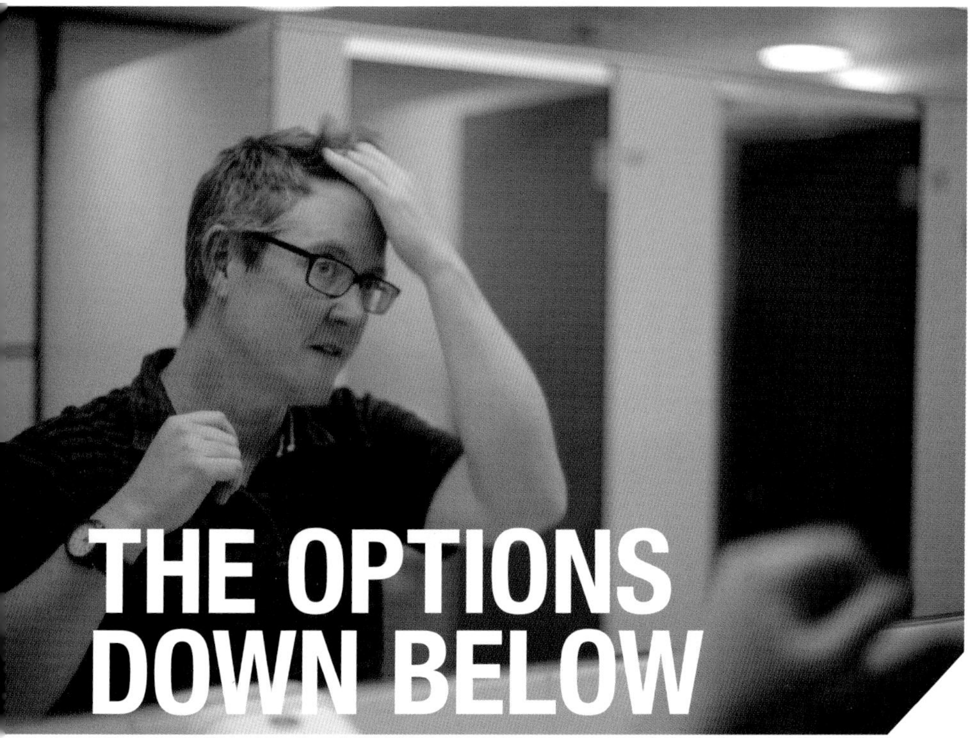

THE OPTIONS DOWN BELOW

There are a number of things you can do to change how your genital area looks and works. This section covers the surgical and non-surgical options.

WHAT ARE THE NON-SURGICAL OPTIONS?

Some trans man like to 'pack' – this means wearing a prosthetic penis in their pants that gives a realistic bulge down below.

There are a large range of 'packers' available. At the expensive end there are some which can be stuck on with surgical glue and are very realistic to look at, with 'veins'. With some you can 'pack and pee' standing up. There are also less expensive 'pack and pee' cocks which are more affordable with less detail on them.

If you can't get to grips with a 'pee' device, there are other options. Cheap packers can be bought through sex toy stores. These can be fixed by a harness but a lot of people prefer using a 'cock sock' or 'packer pouch' to put the cock in which sticks to the inside of your underwear with Velcro. If you're

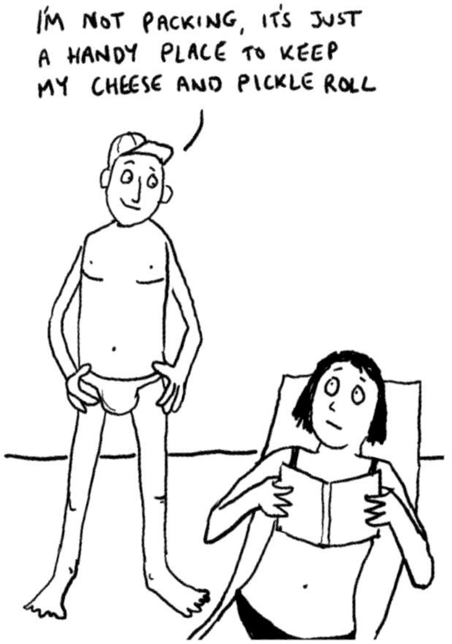

broke, rolled up socks can be quite an effective packer as well.

Some are not bothered about packing but like to have a 'stand up and pee' device handy for camping or long walks in the countryside. Some of these have a cup which is put over the outer labia and others resemble a small medicine spoon which is inserted in the front of the vagina just below the pee hole.

Different designs work for different folk – but they all take a bit of practice to use so try one out at home in the shower first!

DO I NEED TO HAVE A HYSTERECTOMY/ OOPHERECTOMY?

A hysterectomy is a surgical procedure to remove the womb (uterus). Oopherectomy removes the ovaries and is normally done at the same time.

The advantage is that you won't need smear tests anymore and there will never be the fear of getting 'breakthrough bleeding'. Plus, although there is little evidence of an increased risk of cervical or ovarian cancer for those who have been on testosterone a long time, it is still a risk.

Some also find it a relief to get rid of their ovaries and uterus.

If you wish to have lower genital surgery in the future, you may want to speak to your surgeon about the best method to use as some methods for a hysterectomy may impact on later lower surgery options. Some people have hysterectomy at the same time as they have genital surgery.

IF I HAVE A HYSTERECTOMY, CAN I STORE MY EGGS?

Yes. Ideally egg storage should be considered before beginning testosterone.

If you have already started testosterone, it would involve coming off testosterone and being given hormones to stimulate the ovaries. The eggs will then be taken from the body under anaesthetic. This takes a period of months and involves lots of poking and prodding around internally. Egg storage is not as successful as embryo storage and then you would have to find a sperm donor and a surrogate.

WHAT DOES HYSTERECTOMY INVOLVE?

The preferred hysterectomy method for trans men is the laparoscopic hysterectomy coupled with removal of the ovaries and fallopian tubes (salpingo-oopherectomy). This is because this method leaves no visible scars whereas an abdominal hysterectomy leaves a scar on the abdomen. The laparoscopic method also has a faster recovery time than an abdominal hysterectomy.

The organs are removed via the vagina with the assistance of tiny cameras inserted through small holes in the lower abdomen. These leave tiny scars which disappear quite quickly.

WHAT ARE THE RISKS?

The surgeon will go through all of these with you but the main risks are puncture of the bladder or bowel, blood clots on the legs and/or heavy bleeding.

WHICH WARD IN THE HOSPITAL WOULD I GO ON?

This should be your choice. Some prefer to go on to a men's ward or a side room on either the men's or women's ward. The advantage of being on a women's ward is that if there are complications, the experts will be there.

Other people on the ward need not know that a guy is there if it is managed properly – for example, having a dedicated team of nurses allowed into the room, and not having your full name on the door.

I'VE GOT A JOB – HOW MUCH TIME WILL I NEED OFF WORK TO RECOVER?

Like all surgery, your recovery will be easier and quicker if you have a healthy diet and don't smoke.

If you have a laparoscopic hysterectomy you will stay overnight (four nights if you have had abdominal hysterectomy.) You will be discharged once they have removed the catheter and you have had a pee.

You will need to be picked up from the hospital and take time off work – around four weeks if you have the laparoscopic surgery and up to eight if you have had abdominal surgery. You won't be able to drive for about three weeks.

WHAT ABOUT OTHER FORMS OF EXERCISE?

You will have to avoid any strenuous exercise – particularly heavy lifting for three months.

HOW ABOUT SEX?

You can masturbate around two weeks after surgery but if you have penetrative vaginal sex leave this until six weeks after surgery.

I'M NOT SURE ABOUT HAVING LOWER SURGERY

You should never feel pressurised into having genital surgery, by anyone, ever. It is your body and your choice – not anyone else's decision. You should make sure that you are fully informed about all your choices before making any decision.

Having lower surgery may increase your self confidence, but doesn't guarantee an instant change in your relationship or sex life. It helps to know your body and how your own sexual satisfaction works without lower surgery.

Some people leave it for many years until they have decided what they want. Some live a perfectly happy life without ever having lower surgery. Others can't wait to have it. It's your call. GIRES have produced a detailed guide to lower surgery (see page 65).

LOWER SURGERY IS JUST ANOTHER SURGERY, RIGHT?

No. Genital surgery is very different from having top surgery or even a hysterectomy. This is because it usually involves having work done on your plumbing (your urinary system or waterworks) and may affect how you feel sexual sensation. For most procedures it involves a series of operations, each with their own risks, and, if you have a job, lots of time off work to recover.

SO WHAT ARE THE OPTIONS FOR LOWER SURGERY?

There are two main types of lower surgery with options within these. The two main types are metoidioplasty – page 32 – and phalloplasty – page 33. Most surgeries are 'customisable' to a certain degree – for example, you can choose not to have a vaginectomy or urethral lengthening.

You need to think carefully about your choices. If orgasm for you is primarily located within the vagina, you may not want to have a vaginectomy. There are lots of possibilities so before you visit your surgeon, prepare a list of issues that you wish to discuss.

WHAT ARE THE RISKS WITH THE WATERWORKS HOOK-UP?

If you have your waterworks hooked up there are significant risks of leakage (fistula) – usually from the join of the existing urethra (pee tube) to the new one. There is also significant risk of narrowing of the new urethra (called a 'stricture') making it difficult to fully empty the bladder. Both require further surgical procedures. Sometimes hair may grow in the new urethra. Talk to your surgeon.

Regardless of whether or not you have your waterworks hooked up, you will leave hospital with a catheter and bag on your leg – bring trackie bottoms.

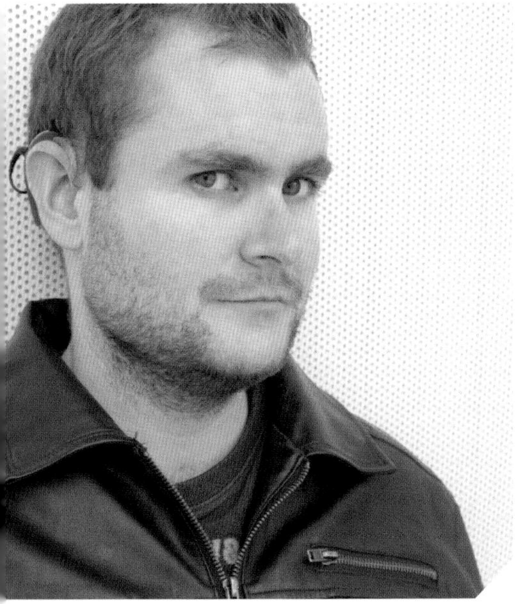

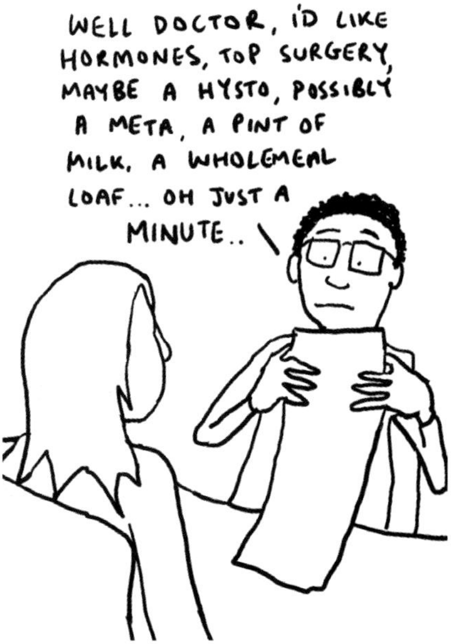

METOIDIOPLASTY

This surgery is recommended for those who are happy with their clitoris/micro penis growth with testosterone and those who tend to be slimmer. This surgery makes use of the growth of the clitoris/micro penis. The ligament that holds it down is cut so it is 'released' and the skin around that area can be pulled up so the position of the micro penis is higher. Skin from the inner labia can be attached to make the micro penis 'fatter'.

In addition, the outer labia may be used to form a scrotum and, in the second stage of the operation, silicone testicular implants are put in.

What about the plumbing?

If you have the 'full works' you will get your waterworks hooked up using 'urethral lengthening' (making the passage down which you pee longer). The tissue used for this usually comes from the vagina or the side of the mouth. Some surgeons will recommend having the vagina removed – a vaginectomy. But you can talk to your surgeon about alternatives if you do not want this.

What about sexual sensation?

This should remain the same – but as with any surgery there is a risk of loss of sensation.

Have I got options?

Yes, it is your body. If you don't want the plumbing done you don't have to. You can also keep the vagina if you wish to.

What's good?

> No visible scars on your body

> The micro penis looks and behaves largely like a penis: you get erections – even 'morning glory'! – although you won't ejaculate.

> May be able to pee standing up

> Less time off work.

What's not so good?

> Not as big a bulge in your pants

> May not be able to penetrate anyone with the micro penis

> Some find they cannot pee standing up without pulling their pants down so can't use urinals.

PHALLOPLASTY

Phalloplasty uses flesh from other parts of the body to make a penis. As several operations are needed with around three months between each, it can take nearly two years not counting complications. The 'abdominal flap' option uses skin from the abdomen as the donor site and the 'forearm flap' option uses skin from the forearm. But there are also new variations coming on which, if you are considering phalloplasty, the surgeon will discuss with you.

ABDOMINAL FLAP PHALLOPLASTY

Before this operation you usually have the hair around the lower abdomen removed through laser treatment or electrolysis – this may mean a few trips to a hair removal clinic beforehand. The surgeon may ask you to put on a little weight around this area to give them more to work with. (If you have a bit of a tummy anyway you are probably good to go!)

A rectangular skin flap from across the abdomen is used to form the penis. The micro penis can be buried in the base or left as it is. You may find it more difficult to masturbate to orgasm, if the clitoris is buried.

This method is usually a four stage job but you don't have to have all stages:

> formation of the penis

> formation of urethra (optional)

> waterworks hook up, testicular implants and glans shaping

> insertion of the prosthetic rod(s), and the removal of a testicular implant which is replaced with a pump, which enables you to achieve an erection.

What about the plumbing?

With this method you can get your waterworks hooked up in a separate operation using skin from your inner forearm or vaginal or labial skin to extend the urethra along the base of the penis.

What about sexual sensation?

There may not be much sexual sensation directly on the penis, though many get a sexual sensation from the clitoris underneath. You should be aware that having a vaginectomy can remove one of the major sites of orgasm.

What's good?

> Less visible scarring. (The scar on your lower abdomen is easily covered by your underwear.)

- No skin graft needed on the 'donor' site if you are not having urethral lengthening
- New phallus may be big enough to take two prosthetic rods, so you will be able to penetrate during sex
- If you have had the waterworks hook up, you will be able to stand and pee, though possibly not at a urinal.

What's not so good?

- May not look like the penis of someone assigned male at birth
- Size of the phallus can vary considerably, it may be short and stubby, or it may be quite thick and need to be 'trimmed' at a later date
- See box on waterworks on page 31.

FOREARM FLAP PHALLOPLASTY

Before this operation you usually have the hair around the forearm removed by laser treatment or electrolysis – if you are right handed it will be your left arm. Again this may mean a few trips to a clinic beforehand.

Skin is taken from the forearm along with an artery, veins and nerves which are connected up at the new site. Skin from the buttocks is used as a graft onto the forearm. The clitoris can be buried in the base of the penis or left as it is.

This is a three (or more) stage job but you don't have to have all stages:

- Formation of the penis and formation of urethra
- vaginectomy and waterworks hook up
- testicular implants and glans shaping
- insertion of the rod to get erections with 'penile prosthesis'.

What about the plumbing?

You can get your waterworks hooked up – 'urethral lengthening'. All the inner labia can be used to create an extension of the urethra into the central cylinder of the phallus enabling you to pee through the phallus.

What about sexual sensation?

Many people report having more sexual sensation with this technique. However, it can take years for the nerves to recover.

You should be aware that having a vaginectomy can remove one of the major sites of orgasm. You should also be aware that embedding the clitoris inside the base of the penis may make it far more difficult to have an orgasm, even from masturbation.

What's good?

- Many guys feel the results look better than the abdominal flap method
- May have sexual sensation directly on the penis
- May be able to penetrate
- Will be able to stand and pee from the end of your phallus.

What's not so good?

- Very noticeable scar on your forearm and a risk of nerve damage to your arm
- May only be possible to insert one prosthetic rod into the phallus so getting the phallus hard enough for intercourse may be difficult.
- More recovery time needed (including about 10 weeks off work)
- See box on waterworks on page 31.

ANY OTHER TIPS?

Whichever operation you choose, you will leave hospital full of antibiotics with a course of antibiotics to follow. Arrange for someone to escort you home from hospital and make sure you have friends to check in with you.

If you are having phalloplasty, take trackie bottoms to wear home as you will have lots of padding around your penis.

Make sure you have lots of food in at home for your return as you won't be shopping for a while. Get lots of fresh fruit to help your body get the extra vitamin C it needs to heal and eat lots of bio – 'live' – yoghurt to put some probiotics back into your body. Make sure your blood sugar is well controlled, especially if you're diabetic, as high or low blood sugar slows healing.

Whatever operation you choose, this is a big undertaking and a shock to the body so do not smoke. Anything! Smoking greatly increases risk of loss of phallus as nicotine constricts the blood vessels.

You have a much better chance of healing well and having fewer complications if your diet is as good as it can be.

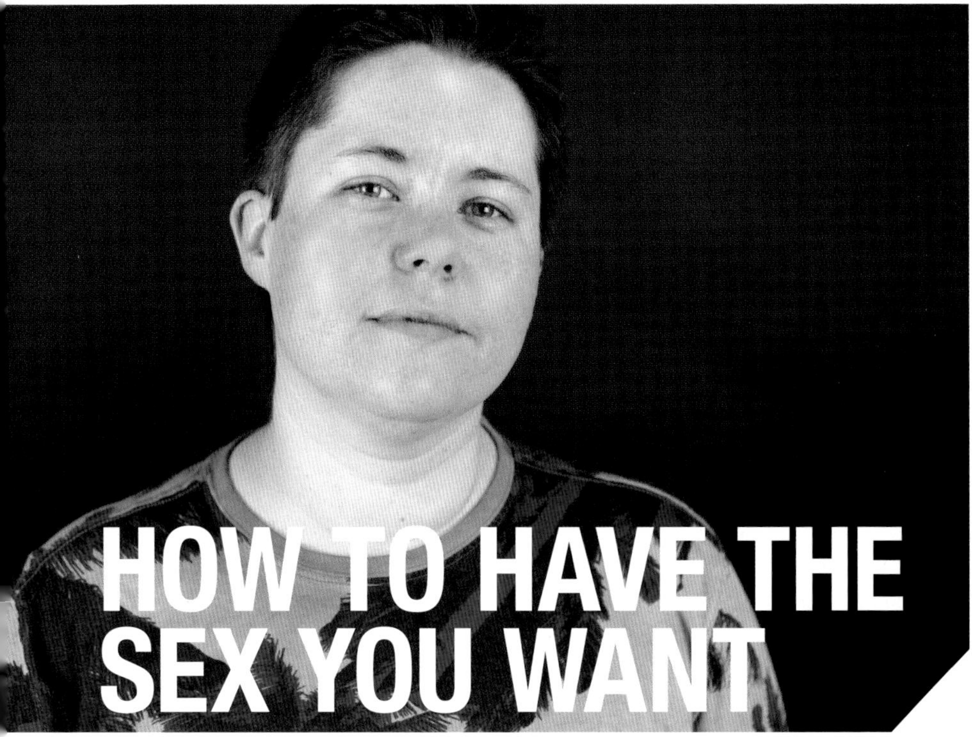

HOW TO HAVE THE SEX YOU WANT

Good sex is about choice whatever our gender identity. This includes the choice not to have it. This section looks at how trans men can enjoy better, safer sex.

Sex can feel great and exploring this with a new confidence or changing body can be very exciting. Lots of trans men feel very comfortable with their bodies before any kind of transition; others come to enjoy them once they start to feel a little different, maybe after hormones or surgery.

Occasionally sex can bring up feelings and emotions about our bodies that can be hard to deal with. That's fine. You can go slowly if you want. It's also fine not to be interested in sex at all. Sometimes we can feel great when we start something, but that changes as things move on. It's different for all of us and if it feels uncomfortable it's OK to say no at any point.

What's important is that you feel confident you are doing what you enjoy and what you want to do. You shouldn't feel pressured into doing something that makes you feel upset, unsafe or uncomfortable. Have fun exploring what you enjoy and what makes you feel good.

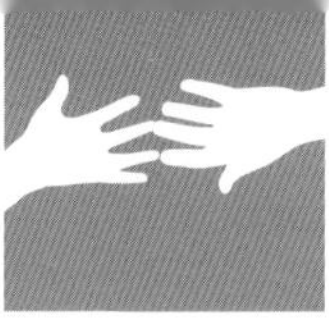

I WANT SEX, BUT I DON'T KNOW WHAT.

Before you get into a sexual situation think about what you definitely don't want to do (hard limits), what you might do with the right person or in the right situation (soft limits) and what you definitely do want to do. Think about things you might want to try out or experiment with, or the things that you can and can't physically do. Knowing this beforehand makes it much easier to negotiate or explain what you want before the pressure is on.

HOW CAN I TALK ABOUT WHAT I WANT?

Communication is key. Think about what language you feel comfortable using for your body parts and let your partner(s) know. Tell them what you enjoy and also listen to what they might want to do.

Of course, you may not be in a situation where you can talk about these things (such as in a sex club or sauna) but we can communicate in more subtle ways. Moving someone's hand can be a way of saying you do or don't want someone touching you in a certain place.

Nobody is expecting PowerPoint presentations or lengthy lists to compare (although go ahead if that's what turns you on!). Discussing things with your partner(s) means that everyone has the same understanding of what everyone wants and means.

WHAT DO YOU MEAN BY 'SAFE'?

Sometimes we may not fully understand the risks we're taking so it's important that you know what they are, how to reduce them and think about the consequences of your actions. Being safe isn't just about sexually transmitted infections (STIs) but also about your emotional wellbeing and physical safety.

Sometimes risk can be exciting – for example, some people like to have sex in more public spaces. It's important to know what the risks are so you can make a conscious choice. The factsheet 'Cottaging And Cruising: Your Safety, Your Rights And The Law' from Galop in London gives more information (see page 67 for details of Galop).

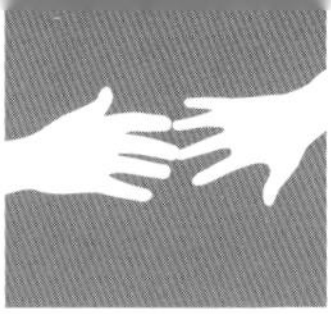

HOW DO I PROTECT MYSELF FROM SEXUALLY TRANSMITTED INFECTIONS (STIS)?

Both social and medical transition can cause changes to the way you experience sex and sexuality, presenting you with many new and enjoyable experiences. Having sex that feels good is important. So is ensuring you are protected from sexually transmitted infections (STIs) and HIV.

There are various activities which can leave us vulnerable to STIs. The highest risk is unprotected anal sex or unprotected vaginal sex. Fortunately, there are many ways we can protect ourselves. These include using a condom for anal or vaginal sex, using a dental dam for oral sex, and using water-based lubrication to decrease the chances of condoms or dams tearing.

If you've recently had surgery, make sure it's healed, that you won't pull scars, do internal damage or open wounds and that there's no risk of the area getting infected. If you're unsure, then speak to your surgeon or doctor.

SHOULD I HAVE CERVICAL SCREENING?

For anyone with a cervix, who is over 25, it is important to undertake a cervical screen ('smear test') to check for abnormalities which might indicate cervical cancer. NHS guidance says those between 25 and 64 should be tested regularly (although it is possible for people of all ages to develop cervical cancer). Women in the UK are automatically added to a register and are notified by their GP of when to screen. However, for people who have changed their gender marker to 'M' on their GP details, it is important to speak to your doctor, as you may not be invited to screening automatically.

The test isn't designed to detect cancer, but to identify abnormal cells on the cervix. One in 20 people will have a test that shows abnormal cells, but this doesn't mean that you have or will get cancer. Most cells go back to normal on their own but some cells will need to be removed.

We understand that as a trans person the process might not be easy but it could save your life, so a few minutes of discomfort is worth it. If you find out later that you have cancer, you're likely to have to go through far more invasive procedures so a 'smear test' can be the best way to look after your health.

SHOULD I GET TESTED FOR STIS AND HEPATITIS?

There are many types of sexually transmitted infections (STIs) and other infections that can affect our health and genitals including chlamydia, herpes, thrush, gonorrhea, syphilis and pubic lice. You can get tested for all of these

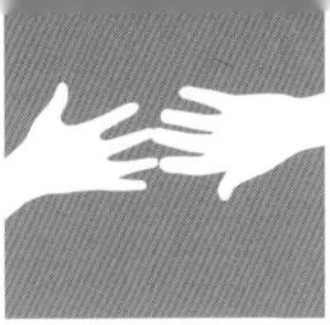

and HIV at a sexual health clinic. Most clinics will also provide cervical screening to check for signs of cervical cancer.

Getting tested can feel scary but it's really important to get tested for your own and your partners' health.

Most infections are easily treated as long as they're caught quickly enough. So if you've had unprotected sex, don't wait for signs that you're unwell, get tested. It is a good idea to get tested regularly. Some STIs don't have symptoms anyway.

Being trans, we may not want to get tested because of a fear of exposing ourselves but these services are confidential and no information will be passed onto your GP unless you request it. Most tests involve testing blood or urine and if swabs are needed, some clinics will allow you to swab yourself. Why not give your local clinic a call to get an idea of how knowledgeable the staff are and find out how they can accommodate your needs.

Even if you're careful and using protection or having sex that's thought to be less risky, it's best to get tested to be sure. The only other way to be sure is not to have sex. You should always consider getting tested before having sex with a new partner.

WHAT DO I DO IF I THINK I MAY HAVE AN STI/HIV?

If you think you may be at risk, then the first thing to do is to get a test done to see whether you have an STI or HIV or not. The sooner you know, the sooner you can get treatment. You're also less likely to pass it onto someone else.

Infections like chlamydia and gonorrhea can be treated with a simple course of antibiotics. However, many STIs do not cause symptoms, so regular check-ups and testing is important.

If you think you may have been exposed to HIV, you can use a treatment called PEP (Post-exposure Prophylaxis) which can stop the virus once it has entered your body. It is a powerful combination of drugs that must be started within 72 hours of exposure and taken for 28 days. It is available from A&E and most sexual health clinics.

WHERE CAN I GO FOR TESTS?

Your doctor can run sexual health and HIV tests or you can go to your local sexual health clinic which is run by the NHS.

Sexual health clinics specialise in sexual health and are confidential (even if you're under 16). You have to give them a name; it doesn't have to be your real one. But make sure you give them the right contact information so they can get in touch about the results of any tests. You may feel embarrassed about the reasons you're there but staff at the clinic will have seen it all before.

Brook offer a service for young people and will be aware of issues that affect young people specifically.

IS THERE A SERVICE THAT UNDERSTANDS TRANS PEOPLE?

If you are worried that staff at a mainstream service may not be aware of your needs as a trans person, CliniQ in London has been created to advise and support trans people and their partners and lovers. It is trans led and all staff are fully trained in trans awareness.
They're able to offer:

> free and confidential sexual health service
> instant HIV testing
> hepatitis B testing and vaccination
> access to liver function testing
> cervical smear testing
> support around sexual abuse
> drug and alcohol support
> counselling
> advocacy
> mentoring.

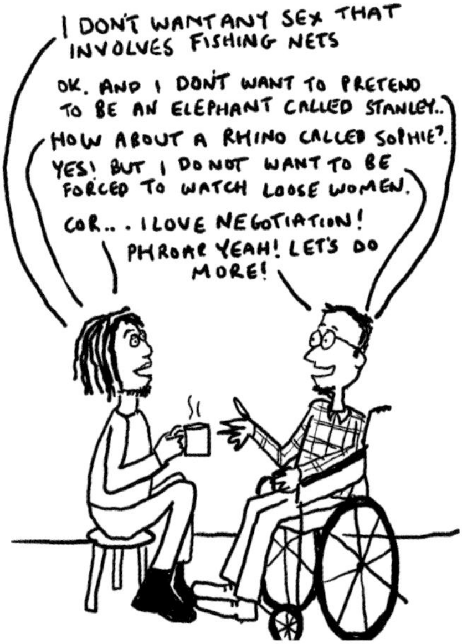

Details on page 67. (There is also Clinic T in Brighton).

WHEN SHOULD I USE PROTECTION?

If the sex you're having involves penetration (this could be a finger, fist, penis/ phallus, either biological, surgically enhanced or shop-bought), think about using a barrier to make it safer. It could be in the form of gloves, a dental dam, a condom or a femidom.

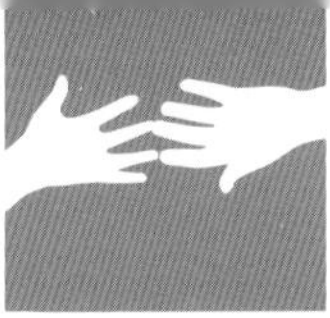

Not only does this reduce the risk of passing on infections, but it also reduces the risk of unwanted pregnancy. Although it is less likely for someone on testosterone to get pregnant, it is possible and if you're not taking testosterone then it's even more of a risk.

If you are trying to get pregnant then you'll need to think about other ways to keep yourself safe, such as sharing sexual histories with your partner, being honest and getting tested for STIs, so you know your own health status.

The anal or vaginal walls are delicate and prone to traumatic injury. Many people on testosterone have reported a further weakening (which could be due to lower levels of oestrogen), resulting in small tears. This means you might bleed more easily, increasing the risk of infection, making it even more important to use a condom, gloves or femidom and water-based lubricant. If you do find that this is an issue, you can speak to your GP who will likely do some tests to make sure nothing else is causing the problem and who can prescribe topical (locally applied) oestrogen to help.

WHAT ABOUT LUBE?

Some people have found that their vagina produces less natural lubricant after starting on testosterone and the anus doesn't produce any. To reduce risks of tearing the delicate skin and to make penetration feel more comfortable, you might want to consider using lube. There are different types of lube available. Water or silicon based lube can be used safely with condoms. Make sure you know which one you are using as silicon-based lube can damage silicone toys and oil-based lube can damage latex condoms.

WHAT ABOUT MY EMOTIONAL SAFETY?

It's really important that you're having the sex you want. Sometimes we challenge ourselves and go outside our comfort zones which can be exciting. But it can be hard too and being aware of that can help. If you start to panic a little, that's fine. Just take a step back and communicate with your partner(s) about what you need. Sometimes talking beforehand about fears can help with this as then you're all prepared for it.

WHAT IF I DON'T WANT SEX OR WANT TO STOP?

It's important that you feel safe and comfortable. You shouldn't feel pressured into doing things you don't want to do or having sex when you're not ready or in the mood. If you change your mind and find that you're not comfortable with something once you've started it, then you have the right to stop. If anyone you're with doesn't respect this, then they're not respecting you and it can be defined as sexual assault or abuse.

There are some trans people who've had sex with someone and felt pressured to do something they don't feel happy or comfortable about but have thought they ought to go ahead with it as they might not get another opportunity ('no-one else will fancy me because I'm trans'). Respect yourself. If someone isn't listening to you and your needs as well, then this may be an unsafe or risky situation.

WHAT IS CONSENT?

The sex you have should be consensual, meaning that you and anyone else participating should have agreed to it. The law says that this should be an active agreement by choice. If you've taken drugs or been drinking you may be at more risk as you are less aware of your surroundings and may have less control over what you do. You may also be more likely to do something you wouldn't do if you were sober.

WHERE CAN I GET SUPPORT FOR SEXUAL ABUSE?

There are many mainstream organisations that can help support people who have experienced sexual abuse, assault or domestic violence. They have resources and experience in supporting people. These services are often local and easy to access and they know the local area and other support that you might benefit from. Some of them are inclusive and knowledgeable of trans issues. Check what is out there. Find out whether anyone else has used them and how they found the service.

ARE THERE SPECIFIC SERVICES FOR TRANS PEOPLE?

There are also a small number of specialist LGB&T support services. They may not be local to you but may be able to offer phone or online support as well as face to face services. You might feel a specific LGB&T organisation is more appropriate for you, as being trans might be an important aspect in your particular situation, and that you need someone who understands this without you having to worry about explaining it. Broken Rainbow and Galop are both trans-friendly and supportive organisations and their details can be found at the back of the booklet.

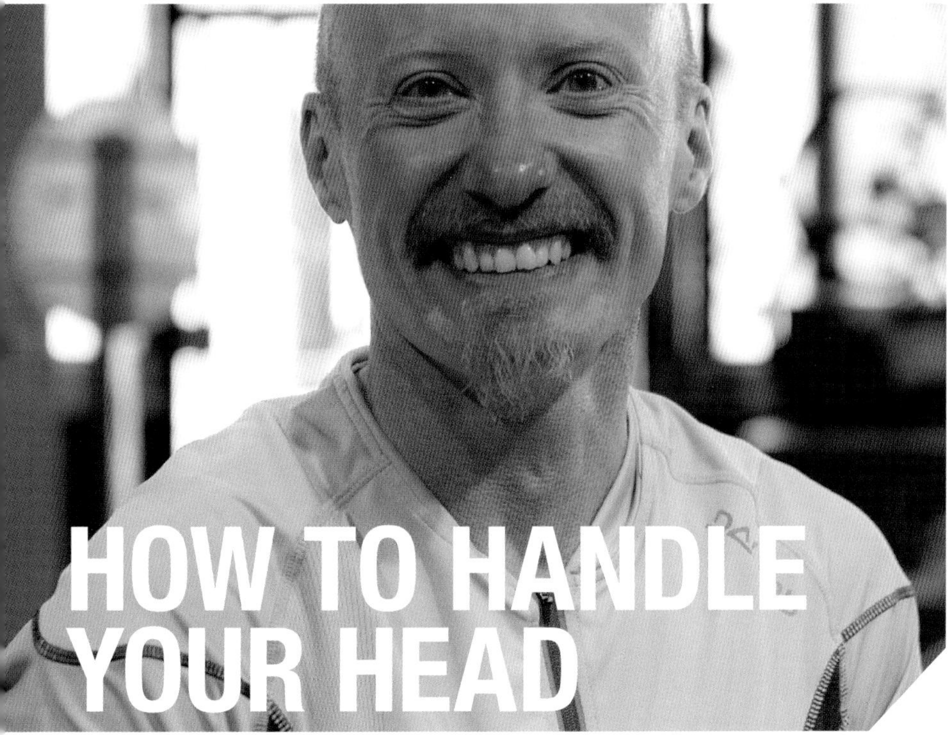

HOW TO HANDLE YOUR HEAD

Anyone can have mental health problems – trans or not.

Just because you're trans doesn't mean that you will have difficulties. In fact, a lot of trans people find that their mental wellbeing improves once they're able to express their gender identity. (In the Trans Mental Health Study 2012, 74% of trans people felt that being able to transition improved their mental health and 81% felt they gained something as a result of being trans or being able to express their gender identity).

Having said that, 84% of those surveyed had had thoughts of suicide at some point in their lives. As trans men, it's as important that we look after our mental wellbeing as it is for anyone else. This section will try to help if you're struggling or need advice.

WHAT DO YOU MEAN BY MENTAL HEALTH?

When we talk about mental health, we're talking about our psychological state, how we feel. One in four people will have mental health difficulties at some point in their life. For some it's dependent on their situation and what's going on in their lives – they may struggle for a short while, for example, after a bereavement – whereas others experience longer lasting or recurring difficulties including depression, anxiety and psychosis.

Mental ill health can affect your life in many ways and can change the way you think, feel and behave. The Trans Mental Health Study 2012 showed that many trans people experience mental health difficulties just like the rest of the population, but that higher numbers of trans people experience stress, depression and anxiety. Sometimes being trans can cause extra stresses and it's important that we're aware of this and look after our mental health.

CAN MENTAL HEALTH DIFFICULTIES AFFECT MY TRANSITION?

It can – and that affect can be both positive and negative – but it shouldn't stop you from receiving treatment. The clinicians at the gender clinic will want to make sure that you are well enough to be able to cope with the process. They will work together with any psychologist or psychiatrist that you may already be seeing.

HOW DO I DEAL WITH PRESSURES TO BE THE 'RIGHT TYPE' OF TRANS PERSON?

As trans people we get all sorts of pressures about how we should be, how our bodies should look and how we should act. For example, your family might have expectations about who you are and what your future looks like. They may have ideas about what being male or female means, which may not fit your view of yourself, or they might not understand a non-binary identity.

Some people feel pressure from gender clinics and worry that they're not trans or male enough. Or they may feel they shouldn't enjoy or like their whole body as it is.

Even pressure from our own communities can exist. People may be told that they should be doing or not doing something in order to fit in, such as having surgery or hormones, or that they should identify or act in a certain way.

If you are finding there are lots of pressures on you, it can be hard to know who you are and what you want to do. The most important thing to remember is to be honest to yourself. There is no wrong or right way to do it. You can go at your own pace and make informed decisions.

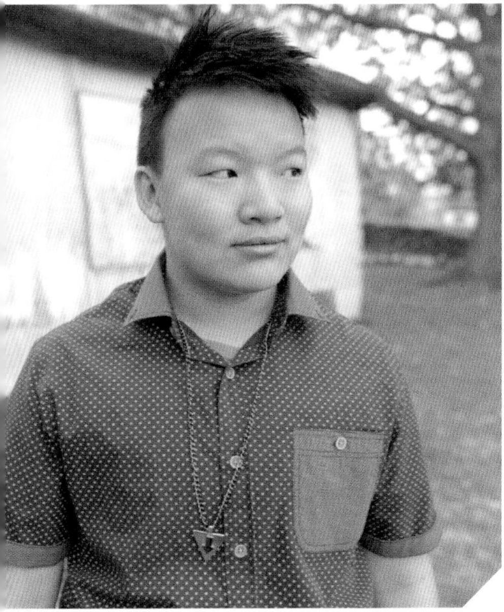

Take time to decide what it is you need to do, how you feel and what's important to you.

Talk to others, read blogs/forums, watch videos and learn about different experiences to help find what is right for you.

Find spaces and friendship groups where you can be free to be you and explore who you are with no pressure to do it a certain way.

Get professional advice. Talking to an experienced and trained counsellor or therapist can help you work out what's right for you.

Many trans men feel that they 'should' have different types of surgeries or hormones because of what is expected of them as men. Similarly, people who identify as non-binary are often expected to be a certain way and to have (or not have, depending on your social circles) medical intervention. There is little understanding of non-binary identities and there can be added pressure to conform to a more 'male' or 'female' presentation or body. It can be confusing for some non-binary people to work out what is right for them as there are fewer resources and information to help you work out what's right for you.

Some people know exactly what they want and need, but some don't. It is really important to remember that if you feel distressed, there is no rush. You will have a better experience long-term if you spend time thinking through your decisions. We make the choices we make with the knowledge we have at the time, so get as much information as you can and try not to give yourself a hard time if you feel confused or uncertain.

Through transition, you may regret some of the decisions you made when you were younger and some of the ways you punished yourself or neglected your health. Think about the future: you may not always have a body that you find hard to live with. Be kind to yourself, give yourself time to adjust and time to look after your health and your needs. Find time to laugh and do the things you enjoy and remember that there is more in your life than just being trans.

HOW DO I KEEP MYSELF MENTALLY HEALTHY?

Being ill or struggling with poor mental health isn't 'bad'. It's part of life. We shouldn't blame ourselves or be ashamed of it. However, there are lots of things you can do to support your emotional wellbeing. (See the Lifestyle section on page 48.)

Eat well – a balanced diet with fresh fruit and vegetables is really important. If you feel low it's easy to reach for fatty, sugary foods. Have a balance of vitamins and minerals.

Exercise – regular, moderate exercise (say half an hour three times a week) helps with mood and anxiety problems. If we feel down we might avoid this, but that just leaves us feeling worse.

Find people to talk with – talking can help a lot. Part of staying happy is sharing the things that are getting to you, which can stop them building up.

Find out what support is out there – if you are struggling because of problems where you are living or you are being treated badly by others, you don't have to put up with it. You can report problems to the police, get in touch with PALS (Patient Advice and Liaison Services) for NHS support, or get help from Citizens Advice Bureau.

Many people have found Mindfulness to be useful in helping us be more aware of what is going on inside and outside of our bodies and in improving mental wellbeing. There are many websites with more information on the benefits and how to do it. There is a link to the NHS website (follow the link to the Men's Health Forum site on page 65).

HOW DO I DEAL WITH STRESS, DEPRESSION & ANXIETY?

It is not necessarily unusual to have a day when you feel low or anxious. It is part of being human. However, if the low mood or anxiety continues and affects your ability to function then it may be that you need outside help.

Think about what makes you stressed – is it certain places, people, tasks or things? Think about how you can manage those situations. Can you make them easier to deal with in some way?

Recognise your achievements – it can be easy to focus on the things that are hard or aren't going so well in our lives. Think about what is good in your life and what you enjoy, are proud of or have achieved.

Take breaks – try not to do everything at once. Take time for you and do things in manageable chunks. You might find it easier to make a list of what needs doing so you can see it and see how you're progressing.

Look after yourself – think about things that make you feel cared for or relaxed, such as having a warm bath or good food. Do the things that you enjoy and make you feel happy. Build in time for these things even if you don't think you feel like doing them.

I FEEL STRESSED OR ILL, WHO CAN I TALK TO?

There is support out there if you're struggling. You are not alone and there are people who can help you. Don't try to deal with it all by yourself, it's OK to ask for support.

You might be able to talk to friends or family and get some support from them. Finding people who understand you and what you're going through or talking to others who have experienced similar things can be really useful.

Your GP will be able to offer support and refer you to a counsellor or your local crisis team. These teams are designed to give urgent help to those who are experiencing a mental health crisis and can support you at home or refer you to other useful services.

National charities like Samaritans, MIND and local organisations and groups can also help. Samaritans are available 24 hours a day to talk to people on the phone and you can also email them. (Details on page 67.)

If you feel that you're at risk of harm or may be putting others at risk right now, go to your local A&E department or contact your GP.

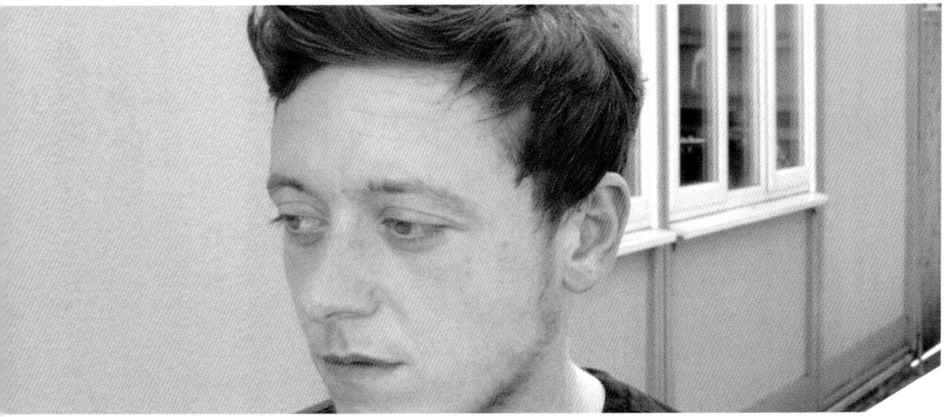

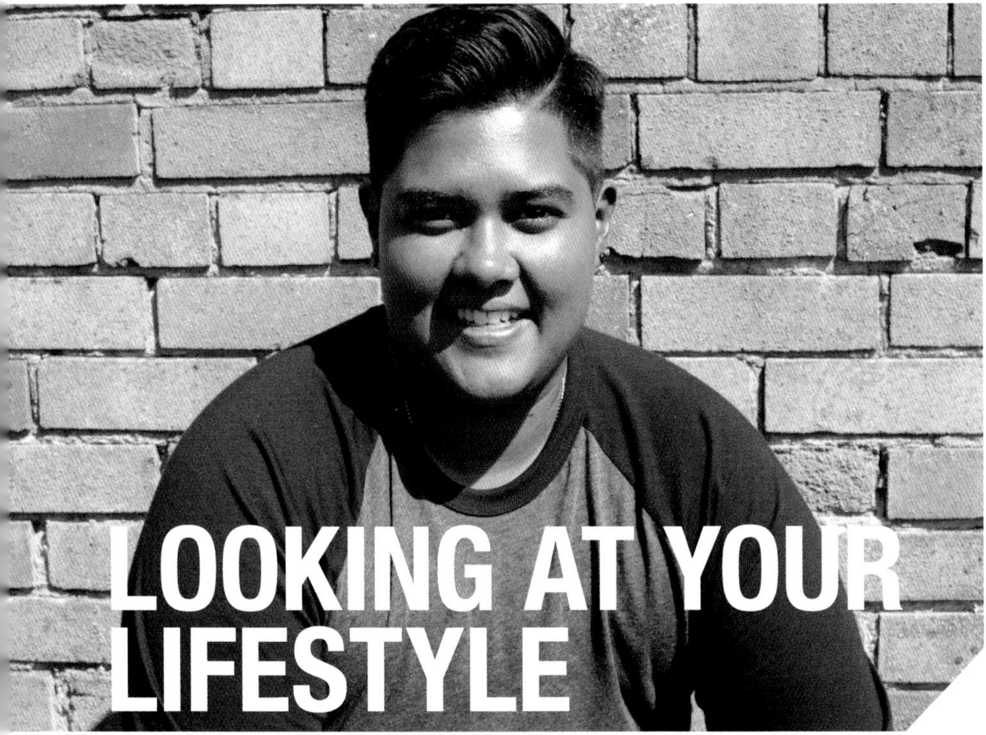

LOOKING AT YOUR LIFESTYLE

Men don't live as long as women. Much of the gap is down to the lifestyle choices we make. This section looks at the small changes that can make a big difference to your health. Look after your body and it should look after you.

I'M HUNGRY ALL THE TIME

If you have just started testosterone you may find that you have an increased appetite and enjoy your food more. You may also find that your fat distribution has changed and you are now storing fat around the waist. This raises the risks of heart disease, high blood pressure, diabetes and cancer. It is important that you make some informed choices about what you eat.

Dieting to lose fat may actually encourage your body to retain calories so it is best to control weight through healthier eating and regular exercise.

Diet also has an effect on your mood and energy levels. Eating small amounts at regular intervals during the day maintains your blood sugar levels and keeps you energised – and less likely to get stressed out or grumpy!

Breakfast is probably the most important meal you can have. It will set you up for the day. Try and avoid cereals that are very high in sugar and salt – read the label on the pack. Porridge is a good healthy filler.

WHAT ABOUT WATER?

We lose water from our bodies as we breathe, sweat and urinate. Drink water – not fizzy pop. Check the colour of your pee – it should be straw/transparent yellow. Any darker than that then you need to drink more.

If you don't like the taste of your tap water, invest in a water filter to keep in the fridge at home.

WHAT IS WRONG WITH SUGAR?

Sugar is not great. It gives you a quick 'hit' and a burst of energy but then you 'come down' off it and have significantly less energy. Avoid sugary drinks like fizzy pop or fruit juice. If you have a sweet tooth, eat whole fruit.

Read food labels. Most pre-packed foods have a nutrition label on the packaging which tells you how much energy, protein, carbohydrate and fat they contain (per 100g and often per serving too). They may also show information on saturated fat, sugars, sodium and salt.

Ingredients are listed in order of quantity. If sugar is one of the first words on a list, it may contain more than is good for you.

Free sugar should be no more than 5% of your daily calories (but aim lower.)

Free sugar is essentially the sugars you have some control over. It includes sugar in manufactured or processed food plus sugar or honey you add to food but excludes sugar found naturally in fruit, veg and dairy. So sugar in an apple doesn't count but sugar in apple juice does (since juice is processed).

Keep the cheesecake as a treat.

EATING DISORDERS

Sometimes we use food to try to take control of our lives and/or bodies. We may overeat, undereat or even starve ourselves. (Sometimes smoking is used alongside.) It may be about punishing ourselves or changing the way our body looks or works. Whatever the reason, it can seriously damage your health (and your transition). Find people to talk to. Get support.

SHOULD I GO FOR LOW-FAT STUFF?

If something is taken out of a food, something else is usually put in. This means foods labelled as 'low fat' or 'no fat' may be high in sugar or sweeteners.

Also when you use a low-fat food you may well eat more. It may be better to stick with the normal 'full fat' food and use less of it.

ARE ALL FATS BAD?

The only really bad fats are trans-fats – fats artificially processed with water to make them spreadable. They're not actually illegal so avoid products that list partially-hydrogenated fat or oil on the label.

Remember though that all fats are concentrated sources of energy (9 calories per gram) so go easy.

When checking labels:

> 3g (per 100g - or per serving if less than 100g) is a LITTLE fat;
17.5g (per 100g) is a LOT of fat

> 1.5g of SATURATED fat is a LITTLE fat;
5g of SATURATED fat is a LOT of fat.

WHAT ABOUT RED MEAT?

Red meat is good for you and full of protein and vitamins but you don't need it in every meal you eat. Guidelines for red meat suggest no more than 90g per day – which is around three slices of pork, beef or lamb. Too much red meat in your diet can increase your risk of bowel cancer.

Fish and chicken are good sources of protein and vitamins as well. So are pulses (chick peas, lentils) soya products or Quorn.

Processed food – packets, ready meals etc – often has added salt, sugar and fat. Cook meals from scratch if you can (and learn if you can't) – that way you know exactly what is going into it.

BUT I LIKE PIZZA AND BURGERS

Your body doesn't have to be a temple but if you regularly fill it with rubbish you will feel rubbish. You can eat burgers and pizza as a treat but not as a regular feature of your diet.

WHAT ABOUT SNACKING?

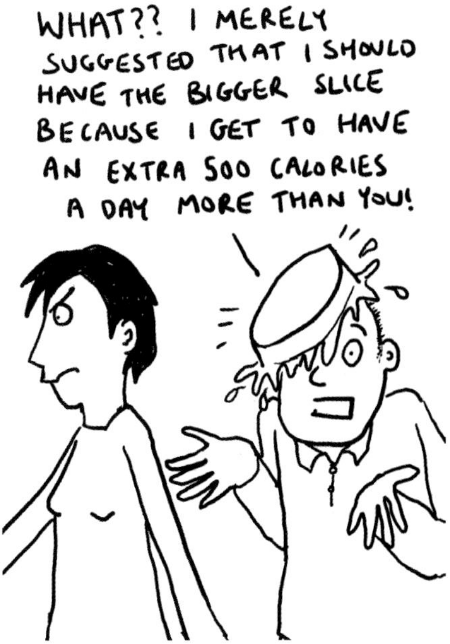

Snacking is no bad thing if you make some healthy choices. Oatcakes are filling and satisfying – and you can get different flavours. Try swapping a packet of crisps for a banana and you will feel fuller longer.

WHAT'S WRONG WITH SALT?

Too much salt can raise your blood pressure. You can add lemon or lime juice to cooking to get the same effect as salt. Ready meals often have a lot of salt so read the label (0.3g per 100g is a little salt, 1.5g a lot).

WHAT'S SO GOOD ABOUT BROWN RICE AND PASTA?

They have more nutrients in them. They are called 'complex carbohydrates' as they take longer to digest giving a nice slow release of energy.

'Refined carbohydrates' found in white bread, white rice and pasta give you a spike of energy which soon wears off. (Check the bread you buy is labelled 'wholewheat' rather than 'brown' – it may be white bread with caramel added!)

I DON'T LIKE FRUIT AND VEG

You probably do but just don't like them overcooked. Try to include them in your meals. You can disguise them – for example by slicing up and chucking them in a stir fry. If you don't like fruit, try a smoothie (but if you are buying a smoothie read the label to check for added sugar).

WHAT IS THE BEST WAY TO GO ON A DIET?

Diets rarely work because when they finish the weight tends to go on again. If you have a healthy diet and take exercise often you shouldn't need to diet.

There is more on food in the Men's Health Forum's man manual 'Eat. Drink. Don't Diet' and on the website.

WHY IS EXERCISE GOOD?

Exercise can lift your mood and contribute to you feeling good about yourself. It can help you lose weight if you need to for surgery and if you are on testosterone you might be surprised how well your body responds. Doing exercise that gets you out of breath makes your body produce hormones (endorphins) that make you feel 'high' and can last for hours afterwards. Even gentle exercise like walking can lift your mood and improve your health.

I DON'T WANT TO BE A 'GYM BUNNY'

You don't have to – there are lots of different ways to take exercise that don't involve joining a gym.

Walking is very good for your health and shedding extra pounds.

Cycling is a cheap form of transport as well as a way of keeping fit. Once you have a bike, helmet and waterproof/visible gear you are all set.

Running is an excellent way of keeping fit – get some decent shoes (not leisure trainers) from a proper running shop who will match shoes to the way you run (your gait). Get a top that absorbs your sweat and you are away.

It is important if you haven't exercised much before – or not for a while, to build up slowly, that way you greatly reduce the risk of injury. If you are unsure, speak to your GP.

Remember to keep hydrated and drink plenty of water – but don't over-do it. For example if you are running for half an hour, you can manage without drinking for that time. You don't need to run with a bottle in your hand and mess up your running style!

HOW DO I CHOOSE A GYM?

Some people find that they haven't got the motivation to exercise alone and find joining a gym helpful. This may be because they like to attend a class at a set time. If you don't like the idea of classes, you can ask a personal trainer at the gym to design an exercise programme to suit you. The advantage of this is that they can show you the correct techniques (form) for doing exercises.

Most gyms are not full of gym bunnies in lycra – you will see all ages, shapes and sizes. It is important to remember that it took a lot of courage for everyone there to go to the gym for the first time.

Visit any gym you're interested in at peak time (usually 6-9pm) and ask yourself a few questions. Is it overcrowded? Is there suitable equipment? Is it clean and well-maintained? Is there somewhere to warm-up/down? What are the changing rooms and showers like? What is the atmosphere like – is it friendly?

Check fees. You don't have to join a private gym. Many local authority gyms are excellent and their staff may have higher levels of gender-awareness.

Try gyms out before joining with a daily or weekly pass. Some offer free trials.

Don't compare yourself with anyone else at the gym. Everyone is different and have their own reasons for being there.

I DON'T FANCY THE MEN'S CHANGING ROOM

Perhaps check out the times when the changing rooms are quieter. (For example, just before or after a class, the changing rooms will be busy.) Or, don't use the changing room – arrive and leave in your gear.

But the truth is men tend to mind their own business in changing rooms. No-one will ask personal questions about you or think you are unusual by changing behind a towel.

If you're worried about scars, remember, many men who are not trans have scars as well and even those who don't can be very modest about their bodies too.

I HAVE A PHYSICAL DISABILITY

Lots of people with a physical disability go to the gym – see our advice above on choosing a gym.

There are about 400 gyms with Inclusive Fitness Initiative (IFI) accreditation which means they're approved by the English Federation of Disability Sport for their accessible facilities, equipment and staff awareness. A trainer at the gym can design a personal programme to suit you.

WHAT ABOUT WEIGHTS?

Doing weight training is one way to get into shape as well as lose weight and increase bone density, reducing the risk of osteoporosis.

It is important to lift weights the right way – it prevents injury and also ensures that you are targeting the muscle correctly. If you are a member of a gym, one of the trainers can show you how to lift the right way (form).

Don't compare the weights you are lifting with others – you should have your own personal goals relative to your body weight. So if you are 5' 2" and weigh 12 stone, you will not be lifting the same weights as someone 6' and weighing 15 stone. However, if you are shorter, you will tend to put muscle on faster than someone taller. This is because long limbs give more leverage (range of motion) when lifting making it harder to build muscle!

I THINK I MIGHT TRY WEIGHTS AT HOME FIRST

To do weights at home, you could buy your gear second hand. (The best time is spring after people have given up on new year resolutions and want to get rid of equipment!)

It is important to develop a good technique (form) for weights or you will injure yourself. Get someone who knows how to do it to give you a session. You can watch video tutorials online for correct form – see www.bodybuilding.com

Remember it is better to lift a lighter weight for more repetitions correctly than to use a heavier weight with bad form and injure yourself.

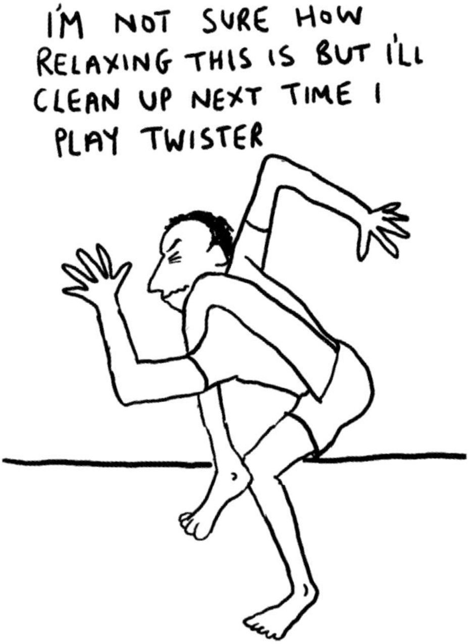

HOW DO I MAKE EXERCISE MORE FUN?

Studies have found that music can have an impact on your performance and give you a boost when your energy is flagging. Find music compilations to accompany different exercises online. Or dig out your favourite tunes and have a smile on your face while exercising!

The most important thing is to find something you enjoy and stick with it. There is no point in flogging yourself at a spinning class at the gym if you don't like spinning!

And remember don't set yourself up to fail. People who tend to stick with exercise usually do it twice a week rather than those who set themselves a goal of four times a week.

WHAT ABOUT SMOKING?

There is no safe level for smoking and you will do your body a big favour if you stop.

If you are intending to have any surgery, many surgeons are reluctant to operate on smokers. This is because smoking can cause breathing problems during the operation, blood clots and infections.

If you have had surgery your body will recover a lot quicker if you are not smoking and wounds will heal better – give your body a chance!

WHAT DOES SMOKING DO TO YOUR BODY?

You probably know that smoking starves your body of oxygen and puts poisonous chemicals in your bloodstream but for trans men who are on testosterone, smoking thickens your blood – increasing the risk of blood clots and raising blood pressure (all of which the testosterone is already doing).

When you give up smoking you will have more energy, you will feel healthier as your body recovers, you will find that exercising will be much easier and you will save money.

There is lots of help out there to help you quit. Your local stop smoking service can offer support including a quit kit, email support and apps. For more information visit: www.nhs.uk/smokefree

WHAT ABOUT E-CIGARETTES?

Although 'vaping' is significantly less harmful than smoking tobacco, that doesn't mean we know it is safe. Whether you get your nicotine through smoking or vaping, it is still highly addictive. Some research suggests you are still at risk of heart disease and damage to your lungs.

WHAT ABOUT BOOZE?

Alcohol is processed by your liver. You need to look after it, especially if you are taking testosterone as this is also processed by your liver – even if you are using testosterone gel.

DO I FOLLOW THE GUIDELINES FOR MEN OR WOMEN?

There are different recommended safe levels for men and women. They reflect the fact that those assigned female at birth tend to weigh less, be shorter and have less water in their bodies than those assigned male at birth.

If you are taking testosterone, your body will usually retain more water. If you are tall and average weight and taking testosterone you may have a higher tolerance than someone who is not on testosterone and is short and underweight. However, we all process alcohol differently based on our genes and metabolisms – for example, if you are from a south-east Asian background, you may be more sensitive to alcohol than someone from northern Europe.

WHAT IS A UNIT OF ALCOHOL?

One unit of alcohol is half a pint of ordinary strength beer. If you like your lagers, they tend to be stronger (around 5%) meaning half a pint will be 1½ units. A large glass of wine is 3 units.

If you have no idea how many units you are drinking per week, keep a diary and add the units up at the end of the week.

HOW MUCH ARE YOU DRINKING?

Large glass of wine (175ml) 15% alcohol	3 units	120-170 calories
Small glass of wine (125ml) 12%	1.5 units	85-120 calories
Bottle of wine (750ml) 12%	9 units	510-720 calories
Pint of beer 5%	3 units	180 calories
Pint of beer 3.5%	2 units	160-170 calories
Single measure of spirits (25ml) 40%	1 unit	60-75 calories

BUT I LIKE HAVING A FEW DRINKS

If you have a few drinks at the weekend eat well beforehand to soak up the alcohol. And alternate an alcoholic drink with a non-alcoholic one – or a lower alcohol one like a shandy.

Give your liver a chance to recover and have at least 3-4 days after with no alcohol at all.

It takes an hour for your body to break down one unit of alcohol unless – and this is the key point if you're out drinking – you've had another drink. If you have another one, your liver has to start processing this one while still working on the other one. Keep drinking and it gets slower and slower. This means that if you get in your car to drive very early the following morning, you may well be over the limit.

Drinking alcohol can affect your mental health and hangovers tend to make you feel depressed. This is because alcohol lowers the levels of serotonin in your brain – a chemical that helps to regulate your mood.

If you are concerned about your drinking, there is more about alcohol and addiction on the Men's Health Forum website. Or see your GP.

WHAT ABOUT OTHER DRUGS?

Many recreational drugs put your mental health at risk as you get a temporary 'high' followed by a 'comedown' where you feel terrible. Regular recreational drug use can make you paranoid, anxious or depressed.

With illegal drugs you are also at risk of getting a criminal record.

WHAT ABOUT LEGAL HIGHS?

Just because something is legal doesn't mean it is safe. (Fags and booze are legal!) There is little 'quality control' for 'legal highs' so you can easily end up taking something which is stronger than you thought, contains unexpected substances or has a different effect to the one you wanted.

Drugs also affect how you behave and you can end up making poor decisions or even ones that put your physical health in danger – like driving under the influence, being in a dangerous situation without being aware of it, or having unprotected sex.

Like alcohol, if you regularly need to get high on drugs, you need to seek help. There is more about addiction on the Men's Health Forum website.

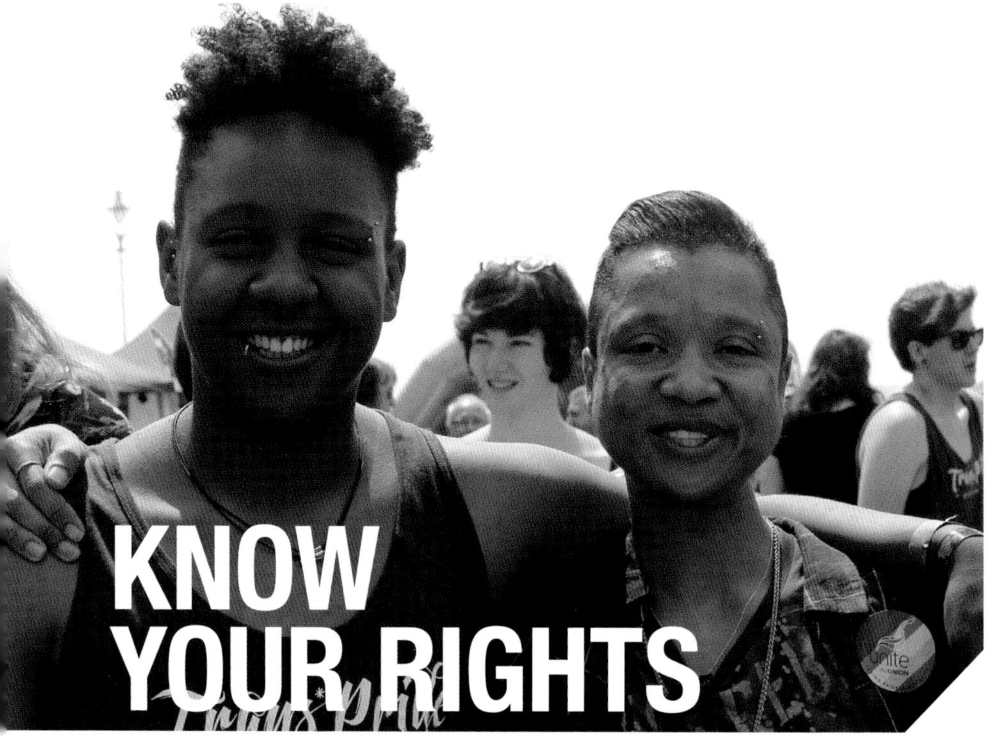

KNOW YOUR RIGHTS

Transition, however you choose to do it, can be a confusing process. This section will try to explain your rights if you do encounter barriers to accessing the options we've discussed.

WHAT IF MY GP IS NOT SUPPORTIVE?

You could ask to see another general practitioner in the same practice. If this does not help, change your GP.

The best people to ask for information about local supportive GPs are local trans support groups. Contact your local LGBT charity for details. If you don't have any local groups, ask on online forums and Facebook groups or see the sources of further information at the end of this guide.

MY GP WILL NOT PRESCRIBE MY HORMONES

Gender dysphoria is a recognised medical condition and specialised consultants in this field have prescribed your treatment.

Your GP should follow the guidance of your Gender Identity Clinic.

You should first complain to your GP and try to get it sorted on the spot. If this does not resolve the problem then ask your GP's practice manager or receptionist for the Complaints Policy and follow the procedure in the policy. If unable to immediately contact you and resolve the issues, your GP must write to you within three working days explaining how they propose to resolve your complaint.

If still dissatisfied, you should send a copy of your complaint to the relevant commissioning body for your GP. (NHS England is the commissioning body for GPs in England while your local Health Authority is your GP's commissioning body in Wales and in Scotland.) You may feel uncomfortable about doing this, and might prefer just to change GPs, but under the Equality Act you are entitled to be treated in a way that is equal with other patients. In other words, your GP should do as they would with other patients and provide the treatment recommended by your consultant.

You should make your complaint as soon as possible after the incident. The time limit for complaints is usually six months from the date of this incident or within six months of you finding out you have a reason to complain (but no longer than 12 months after the event). However, if a hospital or practice is unaware of the matter of the complaint, the six months limit starts from the time they first know about it as long as this is within twelve months of the date of the incident.

I CAN'T USE SUSTANON – BUT MY GP WON'T PRESCRIBE ANYTHING ELSE

If you are allergic to the peanut oil in which Sustanon is suspended or have a very bad reaction at an injection site then you need to look at alternative forms of testosterone treatment. Although only Sustanon is formally licensed for treating trans men, your GP can and should prescribe some other form of testosterone hormone-replacement therapy. (There is more on the various options in our section on hormones – see page 13.)

Some trans men have had their GPs say they are not allowed to prescribe some hormone treatments because of the cost. True, there are big variations in costs – some are about ten times the price of Sustanon – so suggest to your GP that you consider the alternatives together. If your GP is uncooperative, consider changing GP.

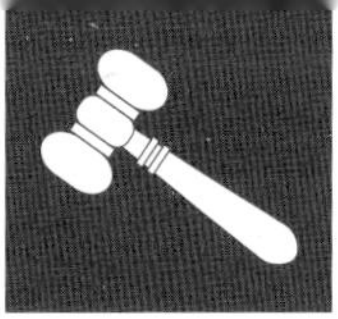

There is guidance from the General Medical Council about prescribing licensed but 'unapproved' hormones ('Prescribing Guidance: Prescribing unlicensed medicines') – full details on page 67.

I'M NOT SURE THE GIC UNDERSTANDS WHAT I WANT

If you are under the care of a Gender Identity Clinic (GIC), remember this is your transition and your choices. Don't get talked into something you don't want. If you have gone as far in your transition as you want and your GP is prescribing what you need, you don't need to go to the GIC any more. However, if you wish to return to a GIC at a later date, you will need to be re-referred and be put on a waiting list.

WHAT ABOUT TAKING TIME OFF WORK FOR SURGERY OR VISITING THE GIC?

Under the Equality Act, your employer cannot ask that you take annual leave time or unpaid leave for any part of your treatment.

For example, if you need to attend your GP's surgery for hormone injections, but the nurse is only available during certain times, your employer must allow you the time off for your injections. Your employer should give you the same rights as they would give to any other person whose treatment was similarly restricted to specific times, for example, an employee who needed to take regular time to attend a fertility treatment clinic for blood tests. You should be reasonable too and, wherever possible, attend clinical appointments outside of your normal working hours, just as you might when attending the dentist.

If undergoing gender reassignment surgery, your employer cannot require you to take annual leave or unpaid leave for your hospital stay or recovery time. Again, your employer should treat you in the same way they would treat any other employee who was undergoing necessary surgical treatment. You are entitled to sick pay, either as laid out in your contract of employment, or statutory sick pay.

Of course, different employers have different policies (many public sector employers, for example, allow up to six months of sickness leave on full pay which goes down to half pay after any six months in one year). But under the law, policies need to be consistent and fair – they cannot have one policy for surgery for, say, cancer and another for surgery for gender reassignment.

I DON'T WANT TO BE 'OUT' AT WORK – WHAT SHOULD I SAY WHEN I NEED TIME OFF FOR SURGERY?

Just tell them you are having an operation and need time off for your surgery and recovery.

All they need to know is how much time you will be off. You can ask the hospital doctor or your GP to be vague on your 'fit for work' note. They could write 'abdominal surgery', for example, or 'chest surgery' and not go into any more details. Your employer is not entitled to know the specific details of any treatment, only whether you are fit or not to return to work.

CAN I GET HELP WITH TRAVEL EXPENSES TO HOSPITAL?

If you are on a very low income and/or benefits you can claim back your travel expenses under the Healthcare Travel Costs Scheme (HTCS). Find out what costs you can claim back and collect the appropriate forms from the Gender Identity Clinic.

CAN I GET TREATMENT IF I AM UNDER A SECTION IN A MENTAL HEALTH HOSPITAL?

You are entitled to treatment if you are diagnosed as suffering from gender dysphoria as it is a recognised medical condition. The process may take a little longer as your mental health clinician and the doctors at the Gender Identity Clinic will want to know that you will benefit from the treatments, and that they will not complicate or make worse any mental health problem you may have.

You will have to wait until you are back in the community before you can be signed off for surgery but you are entitled to other gender reassignment treatments like hormones. You have the right to a mental health advocate to support you and ensure you are respected as yourself.

For more information see the good practice guidelines from the Royal College of Psychiatrists listed on page 67.

Transition doesn't stop because of being seriously mentally unwell, but it can delay it. Try to remember it is only a delay.

I HAVE A LEARNING DISABILITY – CAN I STILL TRANSITION?

You are entitled to the same level of treatment as any other person with gender dysphoria. Your support service should read the good practice guidelines from the Royal College of Psychiatrists (particularly Appendix 1, page 32 for the process) – full details on page 67.

MY GP IS SAYING I DON'T NEED A HYSTERECTOMY – WHAT CAN I DO?

Speak their language. Having a hysterectomy is part of what is called in the NHS jargon your 'gender reassignment care pathway'. This means it is part of your treatment. Show your GP the good practice guidelines from the Royal College of Psychiatrists mentioned above and the information for GPs and other healthcare staff prepared by the GICs: Gender dysphoria services: a guide for General Practitioners and others – full details on page 67. Give them a copy of this guide as well!

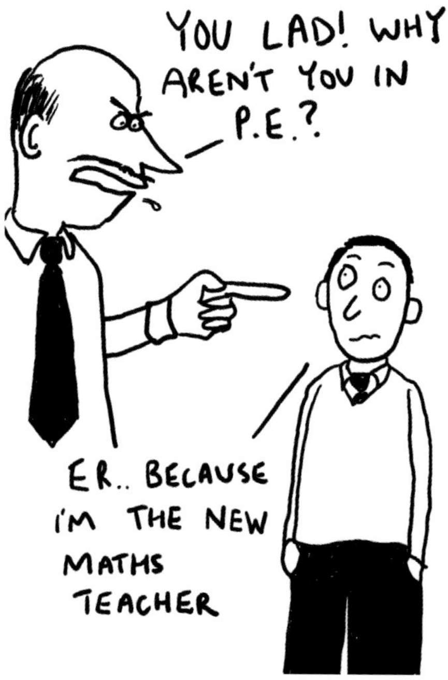

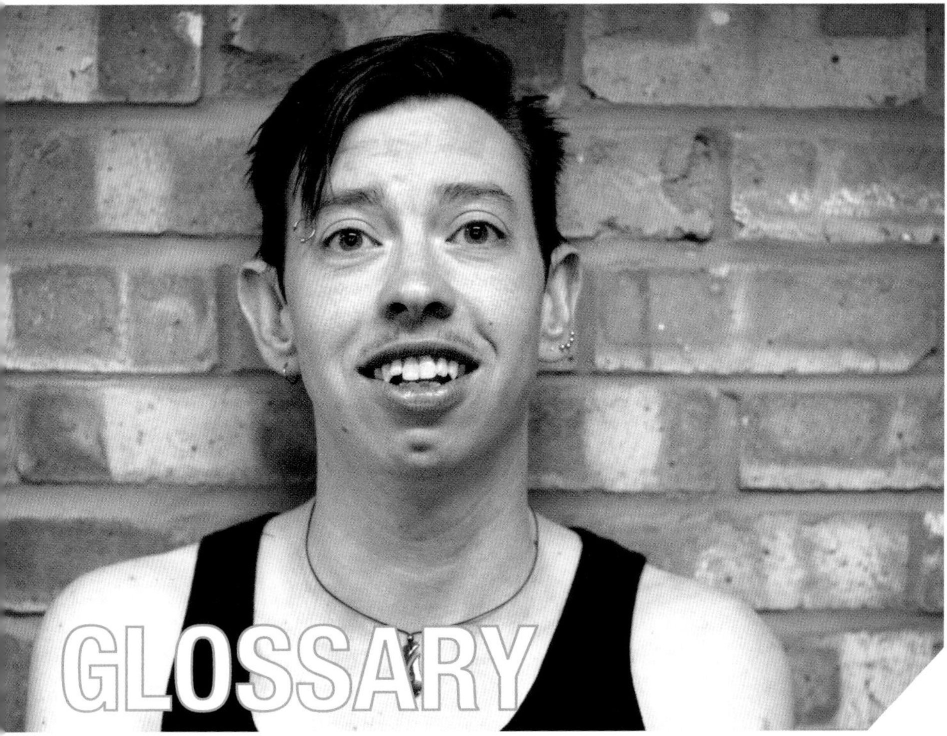

GLOSSARY

Definitions of some of the terms used by doctors and/or the trans community:

AFAB: assigned female at birth.

Affirmed Gender Identity: the gender that a person feels they are.

Assigned Sex: the sex given to a person at birth based on genital appearance.

Gender Affirmation Surgery/Gender Reassignment Surgery: refers to surgical alteration to chest or genitalia, such as phalloplasty/metoidioplasty.

Gender Binary: the (inaccurate) idea that there are only two genders – men and women (and that everyone will fit into this).

Gender Dysphoria: a medical condition (see page 6 for the NHS definition). Some trans men feel this condition applies to them. Some don't.

Gender Identity: a person's internal sense of the gender they are, eg. woman, man, non-binary, fluid etc.

Intersex people: those born with sex characteristics that are not easily classified as what is considered clearly male or female. This could be visually obvious such as genitalia or on a chromosomal/hormonal level. There are many different forms of intersex.

Non-Binary people: those who feel the gender binary of man or woman doesn't fit their gender identity. They often prefer gender neutral pronouns such as they/them. There are many terms for someone who feels like this and it is down to personal preference – for example, genderqueer, genderfluid, bi-gender, poly-gender etc.

Sexual Orientation: who a person is sexually attracted to. This is separate from a person's gender identity.

Trans/Trans*/Transgender: umbrella terms for the whole spectrum of people whose gender identity differs from the sex assigned at birth. This can include any and more of the identities listed. The term is often shortened to trans which is more popularly used, or replaced by gender variant.

Trans man (FTM): a person who was assigned female at birth and identifies as male or masculine.

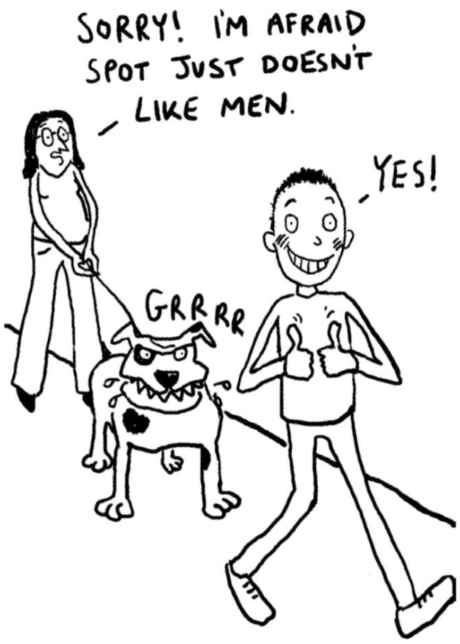

Transition: the process of changing to live life in the affirmed gender role. This is not a simple step but a complex process that can involve many different elements such as medical, legal and social changes.

Transsexual people: those who feel that the sex assigned at birth does not fit with their internal gender identity. They may change their gender role (transition) and possibly have medical treatment, to align their physical characteristics, and their social expression with their gender identity.

GIRES, see page 67, have a more detailed guide to terminology.

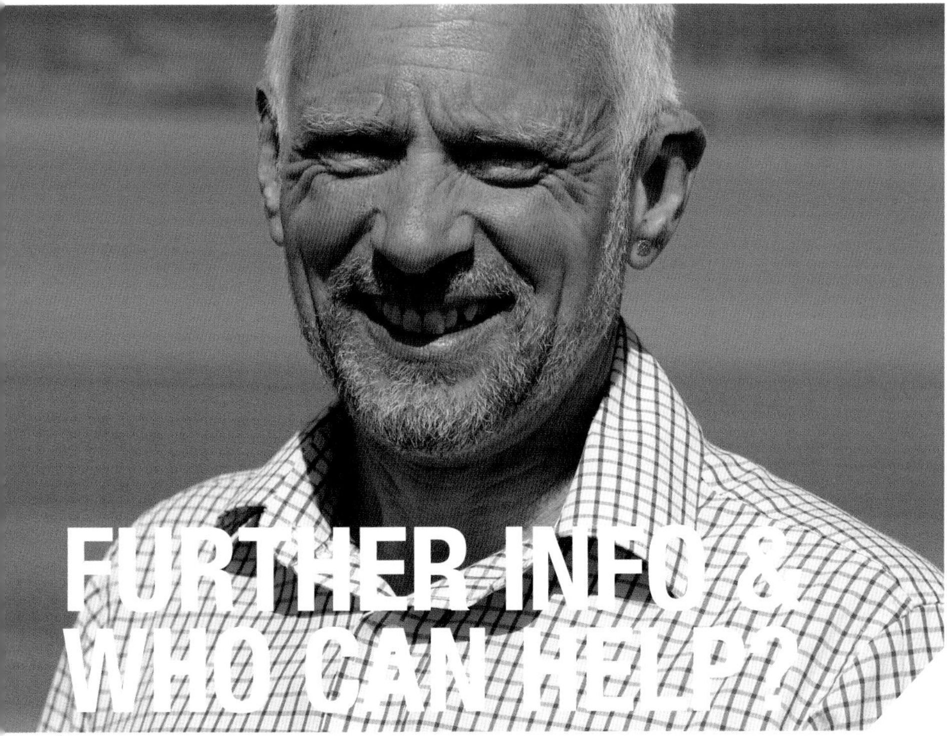

FURTHER INFO & WHO CAN HELP?

The full links for the organisations and publications listed here and many more are on the Men's Health Forum website at: menshealthforum.org.uk/trans

USEFUL PUBLICATIONS

> Living My Life – information for people who currently identify as trans or who are beginning to explore their gender identity (published by the NHS)

> Guide for Parents and Family Members of Trans People in the UK (published by Gendered Intelligence)

> Interim Gender Dysphoria Protocol and Service Guideline 2013/14 – NHS England (September 2013)

> Scottish Gender Reassignment Protocol (published by the Scottish government, CEL 26, 2012)

> A guide to lower surgery for those assigned female, identifying as men, trans masculine, non-binary or non-gender (published by GIRES)

GENDER IDENTITY CLINICS (GIC)

Aberdeen
Royal Cornhill Hospital,
Aberdeen AB25 7ZH
Tel: 0345 456 6000 (Age: 18+)

Belfast
Gender Identity Service, Centre for Psychotherapy, Shimna House, Knockbracken Healthcare Park, Saintfield Rd, Belfast BT8 8BH
Tel: 028 90638854 (Age: 18+)

Edinburgh
Chalmers Sexual Health Clinic, Chalmers Hospital, 2a Chalmers St, Edinburgh EH3 9ES
Tel: 0131 536 1505 (Age: 18+)

Exeter (the Laurels)
Devon Partnership NHS Trust, The Laurels Gender and Sexual Medicine Clinic, 11-15 Dix's Field, Exeter EX1 1QA
Tel: 01392 677077 (Age: 17+)

Glasgow (Sandyford)
Sandyford, 2-6 Sandyford Place, Glasgow G3 7NB
Tel: 0141 211 8130 (Age: 18+)

Inverness
NHS Highland Sexual Health Clinic, Raigmore Hospital, Old Perth Rd, Inverness, Invernessshire IV2 3UJ
Tel: 01463 704202 (Age: 18+)

Leeds (Newsome Centre)
Leeds and York Partnership NHS Foundation Trust, Leeds Gender Identity Service Outpatient's Suite, 1st Floor, Newsome Centre, Seacroft Hospital, York Rd, Leeds LS14 6UH
Tel: 0113 855 6346 (Age: 18+)

London (Charing Cross)
West London Mental Health Trust Gender Identity Clinic, 179–183 Fulham Palace Rd, London W6 8QZ
Tel: 020 8483 2801(Age: 17+)

Newcastle
Northumberland, Tyne & Wear NHS Foundation Trust, Northern Region Gender Dysphoria Service, Benfield House, Walkergate Park Hospital, Newcastle Upon Tyne NE6 4QD
Tel: 0191 287 6130 (Age: 18+)

Northampton
Northamptonshire Healthcare NHS Foundation Trust, Denetre Hospital, London Rd, Daventry NN11 4DY
Tel: 01327 707200 (Age: 18+)

Nottingham
Nottinghamshire Healthcare Trust, Nottingham Gender Clinic, Oxford Corner, 3 Oxford St, Nottingham NG1 5BH
Tel: 0115 876 0160 (Age: 17+)

Sheffield
Porterbrook Clinic, 75 Osbourne Road, Nether Edge Hospital, Sheffield. S11 9BF
Tel: 0114 271 6671(Age: 18+)

Children & Young People (Under 18)
Tavistock and Portman Clinic
The Tavistock Centre, 120 Belsize Lane, London, NW3 5BA
Tel: 020 8938 2030

Knowing Our Identity (KOI), Beechcroft, Foster Green Site, 110 Saintfield Rd, Belfast BT8 6HD
Tel: 02890 638000